MEDICAL TERMINOLOGY
A SHORT COURSE

MEDICAL TERMINOLOGY
A SHORT COURSE

Second Edition

Davi-Ellen Chabner, B.A., M.A.T.

W.B. SAUNDERS COMPANY

A Harcourt Health Sciences Company

Philadelphia   London   New York   St. Louis   Sydney   Toronto

W.B. SAUNDERS COMPANY
A Harcourt Health Sciences Company

The Curtis Center
Independence Square West
Philadelphia, Pennsylvania 19106

Library of Congress Cataloging-in-Publication Data

Chabner, Davi-Ellen,
    Medical terminology : a short course / Davi-Ellen Chabner. — 2nd ed.
     p.   cm.
    Includes index.
    ISBN 0-7216-8124-7
    1. Medicine—Terminology.   I. Title.
    [DNLM: 1. Nomenclature problems.   W 15 C427m   1999]
    R123.C434   1999
    616′.0014—dc20
    DNLM/DLC   98-48477

MEDICAL TERMINOLOGY: A SHORT COURSE   ISBN   0–7216–8124–7

Copyright © 1999, 1991 by W.B. Saunders Company

Printed in the United States of America

Last digit is the print number: 9   8   7   6   5   4   3

To Noonie and Dave
with my gratitude and love for bringing beautiful
Beatrix Bess into our world

and

To Brenda
my long-time friend who shares my new passion
for grandparenthood

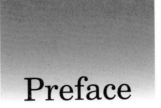

Preface

I am pleased to present the 2nd edition of *Medical Terminology: A Short Course*. In this revision, I have endeavored to preserve the same clarity, practicality, and simplicity that characterized the first edition. For those of you who already use *A Short Course*, you will find its goal essentially unaltered; that is to give an introduction and overview of medical language with emphasis on basic, essential information. For those of you who are new to the text and to my approach to teaching here are some of its important features. *A Short Course* is:

1. A *self-teaching* book with a *workbook-text format*. It follows the teaching method presented in my more complete text, *The Language of Medicine, 5th edition*. You learn by doing; that is, by answering questions, labelling diagrams, testing yourself with review sheets, and practicing pronunciation following the guides in each chapter.

2. A valuable and comprehensive *hospital and medical office reference guide* for use during and after completion of your terminology course. In its Appendices and Glossaries you will find full color diagrams of body systems, explanations of diagnostic tests and procedures, commonly used medical abbreviations AND a handy mini-dictionary of basic medical terms. In this new edition, I have included an English to Spanish Glossary as well.

3. *Easy to read and understand.* I have not presupposed prior knowledge of science or biology. Explanations of terms are worded simply and clearly, and repetition is used to reinforce understanding throughout the text. Answers to each exercise are given directly following the exercise, so that you can conveniently check your responses and learn from the printed answers.

4. *A highly visual and practical* text. I believe in illustrating terminology with simple line diagrams highlighting parts of the body, procedures, and disease conditions presented in the text. We are particu-

larly happy to provide attractive full color illustrations of the body systems in Appendix I along with practical information (combining forms, terminology and pathology) for each system.

New to this edition are *medical vignettes* illustrating medical terminology in the context of stories about patients and *practical applications of terminology* in each chapter. The Instructor's Manual has been expanded to include additional classroom activities, quizzes, crossword puzzles and MORE practical examples of case studies and medical reports.

Medical Terminology: A Short Course is all you need to start your medical career—in an office, hospital, or other medical-related setting. You can work at your own pace or in a classroom setting with the help of an instructor. The combination of "hands-on" visually reinforced learning AND practically useful and accessible reference material will mean success for you in your allied health career!

Most of all, though, I hope that this book excites your interest and enthusiasm for the medical language. I guarantee that, by faithfully working through this book, you will discover the fascination and passion that this subject has ignited in me for over 25 years.

I welcome hearing from you with suggestions and comments, since I am always learning from students and their teachers. My e-mail address is MedDavi @ aol.com. Please communicate, write, and share your experiences with me. Work hard, and have fun with medical terms!

Acknowledgments

Once again, I have had the pleasure of working with the W.B. Saunders staff. As ever, Scott Weaver, my editor, has been essential and utterly dependable. I am grateful to Andrew Allen, Maureen Pfeifer, and Betty Taylor for their unwavering support and confidence in me and my work.

Instructors have written and contributed both to changes in the text and additions to the Instructor's Manual. I am thankful for their suggestions and comments and welcome yours as well. Special thanks go to Kathy Trawick, Little Rock, Arkansas, Ellen Streight, Hamilton, New Jersey, Cindy Correa, Queens, New York, Carole Michael, Charleston, West Virginia, Debi Grienesen, Harrisburg, PA, Pat Bowen, San Diego, California, Rebecca Kelly, Marietta, Georgia, and J.M. Found, Vernon, British Columbia.

My devoted daughter, Dr. Elizabeth Chabner Thompson, composed the medical vignettes in each chapter and patiently stood at the ready to answer any and all of my questions related to medical issues. My loving son, Brandon, effectively took over the financial management of my life and left me time for other pursuits. My staunch and loyal mate of 35 years has always encouraged and supported my passion for teaching and medical terminology. Thanks, Bruce.

Last, but certainly not least, I'm grateful for my two constant canine companions, Eli and Lily, who provide me with endless hours of affection, fun, and love.

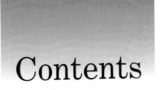

Contents

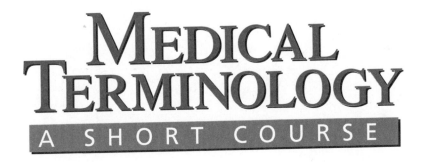

MEDICAL TERMINOLOGY

A SHORT COURSE

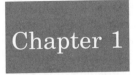

Chapter 1

Basic Word Structure

C H A P T E R   O B J E C T I V E S

- To divide medical terms into component parts
- To analyze, pronounce, and spell medical terms using common combining forms, suffixes, and prefixes

I. Word Analysis

If you work in a medical setting, you use medical words every day. As a consumer and citizen, you hear medical terms in your doctor's office, read about health issues in the newspaper, and make daily decisions about your own health care and the health care of your family. Terms such as *arthritis*, *electrocardiogram*, *hepatitis*, and *anemia* describe conditions and tests that are familiar. Other medical words are more complicated, but as you work in this book, you will begin to understand them even if you have never studied biology or science.

Medical words are like individual jigsaw puzzles. Once you divide the terms into their component parts and learn the meaning of the individual parts, you can use that knowledge to understand many other new terms.

For example, the term HEMATOLOGY is divided into three parts:

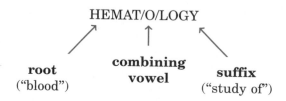

HEMAT/O/LOGY

root
("blood")

combining vowel

suffix
("study of")

When you analyze a medical term, begin at the *end* of the word. The ending is called a **suffix**. All medical terms contain suffixes. The suffix in HEMATOLOGY is -LOGY, which means "study of." Now look at the beginning of the term. HEMAT is the word **root**. The root gives the essential meaning of the term. The root HEMAT- means "blood."

The third part of this term, which is the letter O, has no meaning of its own but is an important connector between the root (HEMAT) and the suffix (LOGY). It is called a **combining vowel**. The letter O is the combining vowel usually found in medical terms.

Putting together the meaning of the suffix and the root, the term HEMATOLOGY means "the study of blood."

Here's another familiar medical term: ELECTROCARDIOGRAM. You probably know this term, often abbreviated as EKG or ECG. This is how you divide it into its parts:

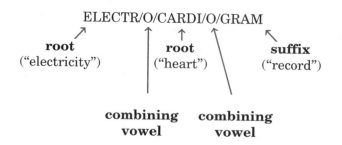

ELECTR/O/CARDI/O/GRAM

root
("electricity")

root
("heart")

suffix
("record")

combining vowel

combining vowel

Start with the **suffix** at the end of the term. The suffix -GRAM means "a record."

Now look at the beginning of the term. ELECTR- is a word **root**, and it means "electricity."

This medical term has two roots. The second root is CARDI-, meaning "heart." Whenever you see CARDI in other medical terms, you will known that it means "heart."

Read the meaning of medical terms from the suffix, back to the beginning of the term, then across. Thus, the entire term means "record of the electricity in the heart." It is the electricity flowing within the heart that causes the heart muscle to contract, pumping blood throughout your body. The contraction and relaxation of heart muscle are called the heartbeat.

Notice the two combining vowels in ELECTROCARDIOGRAM. Looking for the O in medical terms will help you divide the term into its parts. A combining vowel (O) lies between roots (ELECTR and CARDI) and between the root (CARDI) and suffix (GRAM).

The combining vowel *plus* the root is called a **combining form**. For example, there are *two* combining forms in the word ELECTROCARDIOGRAM. These combining forms are ELECTR/O, meaning "electricity," and CARDI/O, meaning "heart."

Notice how the following medical term is analyzed. Can you locate the two combining forms in this term?

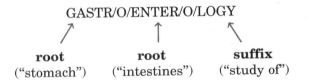

GASTR/O/ENTER/O/LOGY

root	root	suffix
("stomach")	("intestines")	("study of")

The two combining forms are GASTR/O and ENTER/O. The entire word (reading from the suffix, back to the beginning of the term, and across) means "study of the stomach and the intestines." Here are other words that are divided into component parts:

GASTR/O/SCOPE means "Instrument to visually examine the stomach."

combining form ("stomach") **suffix** ("instrument to visually examine")

GASTR/IC means "Pertaining to the stomach." Notice that the combining vowel is *dropped* when the suffix (-IC) begins with a vowel. Words ending in -IC are adjectives and mean "pertaining to."

root ("stomach") **suffix** ("pertaining to")

CARDI/AC   means   "Pertaining to the heart." Again, the combining
vowel is dropped when the suffix (-AC) begins
with a vowel. Words ending in -AC are adjectives
and mean "pertaining to."

root   **suffix**
("heart")   ("pertaining to')

ENTER/ITIS   means   "Inflammation of the intestines." Notice again
that the combining vowel is dropped because the
suffix (-ITIS) begins with a vowel.

root   **suffix**
("intestines")   ("inflammation")

GASTR/O/ENTER/ITIS   means   "Inflammation of the stomach and intestines."
Notice that the combining vowel (O) remains be-
tween the two roots even though the second root
(ENTER) begins with a vowel.

root   **suffix**
("stomach")   ("inflammation")

       root
("intestines")

In addition to roots, suffixes, combining forms, and combining vowels, many
medical terms have a word part attached to the *beginning* of the term. This is
called a **prefix**, and it can change the meaning of a term in important ways. For
example, watch what happens to the meaning of the following medical terms
when the prefix changes:

SUB/gastr/ic   means   "pertaining to *below* the stomach."

prefix
("below")

TRANS/gastr/ic   means   "pertaining to *across* the stomach."

prefix
("across")

RETRO/gastr/ic   means   "pertaining to *behind* the stomach."

prefix
("behind")

Let's **review** the important word parts:

1. **Root**—gives the essential *meaning* of the term.
2. **Suffix**—is the word *ending*.
3. **Prefix**—is a small part added to the *beginning* of a term.
4. **Combining vowel**—*connects* roots to suffixes and roots to other roots.
5. **Combining form**—is the combination of the *root* and *combining vowel*.

Some important rules to *remember* are:

1. *Read* the meaning of medical words from the suffix to the beginning of the word and then across.
2. *Drop* the combining vowel before a suffix that starts with a vowel.
3. *Keep* the combining vowel between word roots, even if the root begins with a vowel.

II. Combining Forms, Suffixes, and Prefixes

Here is a list of combining forms, suffixes, and prefixes that are commonly found in medical terms. Write the meaning of the medical term on the line that is provided. There will be terms that are more difficult to understand even after writing the meanings of individual word parts. For these, more extensive explanations are given. In order to check your work, the meanings to all terms can be found in Glossary of Medical Terms, p. 241.

In your study of medical terminology, you will find it helpful to practice writing terms and their meanings many times. Complete the Exercises in Section III, the Review in Section IV, and the Pronunication of Terms list in Section V, as you begin your study of the medical language.

COMBINING FORMS

Combining Form	Meaning	Medical Term	Meaning
aden/o	gland	adenoma _gland tumor_ -OMA means "tumor" or "mass."	
		adenitis _gland inflammation_ -ITIS means "inflammation."	
arthr/o	joint	arthritis _joint arthritis_	
bi/o	life	biology _study of life_ -LOGY means "study of."	
		biopsy _to view life_ -OPSY means "to view." Living tissue is removed and viewed under a microscope.	

carcin/o	cancer, cancerous
cardi/o	heart
cephal/o	head
cerebr/o	cerebrum, largest part of the brain

carcinoma _cancer tumor or mass_

cardiology _study of the heart_

cephalic _pertaining to head_
-IC means "pertaining to."

cerebral _pertaining to head_
-AL means "pertaining to." Figure 1–1 shows the cerebrum and some of its functions.

cerebrovascular accident (CVA) _stroke_
-VASCULAR means "pertaining to blood vessels"; a CVA is commonly known as a stroke.

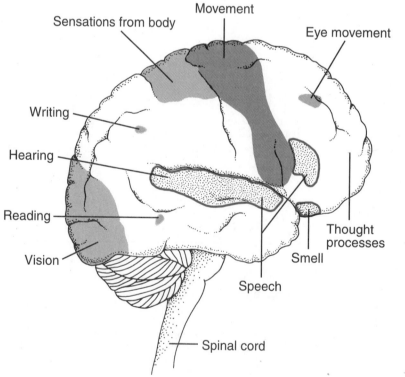

Figure 1–1
The cerebrum and its functions.

cyst/o	urinary bladder	cystoscope _instrument to visually examine_ -SCOPE means "instrument to visually examine." Figure 1–2 shows the urinary tract. A cystoscope is placed through the urethra into the urinary bladder.
cyt/o	cell	cytology _study of cells_
dermat/o	skin	dermatitis _skin infection_
electr/o	electricity	electrocardiogram (ECG, EKG) _record of hearts electricity_ -GRAM means "record."
encephal/o	brain	electroencephalogram (EEG) _record of brain electricity_ This record is helpful in determining if a patient has a seizure disorder, such as epilepsy.

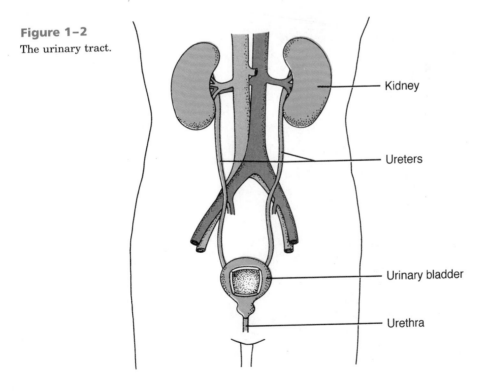

Figure 1–2
The urinary tract.

Kidney

Ureters

Urinary bladder

Urethra

enter/o	intestines (often the small intestine)
erythr/o	red

enteritis _inflammation of intestine_
Figure 1–3 shows the small and large intestines. ENTER/O is used to describe the small intestine and the intestines in general, while COL/O is the combining form for the large intestine (colon).

erythrocyte _cell ~ red_
-CYTE means "cell." Figure 1–4 shows the three major types of blood cells.

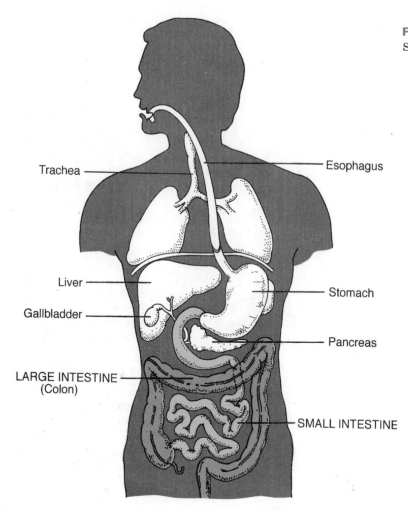

Figure 1–3
Small and large intestines.

Trachea

Esophagus

Liver

Stomach

Gallbladder

Pancreas

LARGE INTESTINE
(Colon)

SMALL INTESTINE

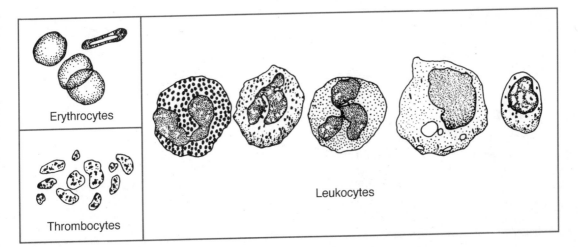

Figure 1–4
Blood cells: erythrocytes (carry oxygen), leukocytes (five different types help fight disease), and thrombocytes or platelets (help blood to clot).

gastr/o	stomach
gnos/o	knowledge
gynec/o	woman
hemat/o	blood

gastroscopy _process of viewing stomach_
-SCOPY means "process of viewing."

diagnosis _state of complete knowledge_
-SIS means "state of"; DIA- means "complete." A diagnosis is the complete knowledge gained after testing and examining the patient. The plural of diagnosis is diagnoses. Table 1–1 shows other plural formations.

prognosis _prediction_
PRO- means "before." A prognosis is a prediction that is made after the diagnosis about the outcome of treatment.

gynecology _study of female disorders_

hematoma _mass of blood_
-OMA means "mass" or "tumor." In this term, -oma indicates a mass or swelling containing blood. A hematoma is a bruise or black-and-blue mark.

TABLE 1–1.   FORMATION OF PLURALS

Consult the Glossary of Medical Terms for pronunciation of all terms.

1. Words ending in **a**, retain the **a** and add **e**:

Singular	Plural	Meaning
vertebra	vertebrae	Backbones
bursa	bursae	Sacs of fluid near a joint

2. Words ending in **is**, drop the **is** and add **es**:

Singular	Plural	Meaning
diagnosis	diagnoses	Determination of the nature and cause of diseases
psychosis	psychoses	Abnormal conditions of the mind

3. Words ending in **ex** and **ix**, drop the **ex** and **ix** and add **ices**:

Singular	Plural	Meaning
apex	apices	Pointed ends of organs
cortex	cortices	Outer parts of organs
varix	varices	Enlarged, swollen veins

4. Words ending in **on**, drop the **on** and add **a**:

Singular	Plural	Meaning
ganglion	ganglia	Groups of nerve cells; benign cysts near a joint (such as the wrist)
spermatozoon	spermatozoa	Sperm cells

5. Words ending in **um**, drop the **um** and add **a**:

Singular	Plural	Meaning
bacterium	bacteria	Types of one-celled organisms
ovum	ova	Egg cells

6. Words ending in **us**, drop the **us** and add **i***:

Singular	Plural	Meaning
bronchus	bronchi	Tubes leading from the windpipe to the lungs
calculus	calculi	Stones

*Exceptions to this rule are viruses and sinuses.

hepat/o	liver	hepatitis _infetion of the liver inflammation_
lapar/o	abdomen (area between the chest and hip)	laparotomy _to cut into the abdomen_ -TOMY means "incision" (to cut into). An exploratory laparotomy is an incision of the abdominal wall to inspect abdominal organs for evidence of disease.
leuk/o	white	leukocyte _white blood cell_ Figure 1–4 shows leukocytes.

nephr/o	kidney	nephrectomy _excision of the kidney_ -ECTOMY means "to cut out," an excision or resection of an organ or part of the body.
neur/o	nerve	neurology _study of nerves_
oste/o	bone	osteoarthritis _inflammation of joints a bone_ Figure 1–5 shows a normal joint and a joint with osteoarthritis.
onc/o	tumor	oncologist _tumor specialist_ -IST means "a specialist."
ophthalm/o	eye	ophthalmoscope _process of viewing the_
path/o	disease	pathologist _disease specialist_ A pathologist is a medical doctor who views biopsy samples to make a diagnosis and examines a dead body (autopsy) to determine the cause of death. AUT- means "self" and -OPSY means "to view." Thus, an autopsy is an opportunity to see for oneself what has happened to the patient to cause his or her death.
psych/o	mind	psychosis _abnormal condition of mind_ -OSIS means "abnormal condition." This is a serious mental condition in which the patient loses touch with reality.

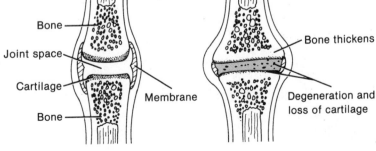

Figure 1–5
Normal joint and osteoarthritis.

Bone

Joint space

Cartilage

Bone

Membrane

Bone thickens

Degeneration and loss of cartilage

ren/o	kidney	renal _pertaining to kidney_

Sometimes there are *two* combining forms for the same part of the body. One comes from Latin, and the other from Greek (REN- is the Latin root meaning "kidney," and NEPHR- is the Greek root). The Greek root is used to describe abnormal conditions and procedures, whereas the Latin root is used with -AL, meaning "pertaining to."

rhin/o	nose	rhinitis _inflammation of nose_
sarc/o	flesh	sarcoma _tumor of flesh_

Sarcomas and carcinomas are cancerous tumors. Sarcomas grow from the "fleshy" tissues of the body, such as muscle, fat, bone, and cartilage, whereas carcinomas arise from skin tissue and the linings of internal organs.

thromb/o	clotting	thrombocyte _cell blood clot_

A thrombocyte (PLATELET) is a small cell that helps blood to clot. Platelets are shown in Figure 1–4.

thrombosis _abnormal cond of clotting_

A thrombus (blood clot) occurs when thrombocytes and other clotting factors combine. Thrombosis describes the condition of forming a clot (thrombus).

SUFFIXES

Suffix	Meaning	Medical Term	Meaning
-al	pertaining to	neural	_pertaining to nerves_
-algia	pain	arthralgia	_pain in the joints_
-cyte	cell	leukocyte	_white blood cell_

-ectomy	removal, excision	gastrectomy _~~excision~~ removal of stomach_
-emia	blood condition	leukemia _white blood cell condition_ Large numbers of immature, cancerous cells are found in the bloodstream and bone marrow (inner part of bone that makes blood cells).
-gram	record	arthrogram _x-ray record of joint_ This is an x-ray record of a joint.
-ic	pertaining to	gastric _____
-ism	condition, process	hyperthyroidism _____ HYPER- means "excessive." The thyroid gland is in the neck. It secretes (makes) a hormone called thyroxine, which helps cells burn food to release energy. See Figure 1–6.
-itis	inflammation	gastroenteritis _inflammation of stomach and small intestine_
-logist	specialist in the study of	neurologist _specialist in the study of nerves_
-logy	study of	nephrology _study of kidney_
-oma	tumor, mass	hepatoma _tumor of liver_
-opsy	to view	biopsy _to view life_
-osis	abnormal condition	nephrosis _abnormal condition_
-scope	instrument to visually examine	gastroscope _instrument to visually examine_

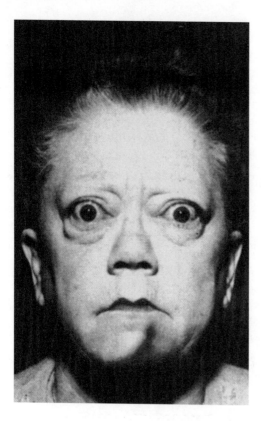

Figure 1–6
Hyperthyroidism: The thyroid gland produces too much hormone and causes symptoms such as rapid pulse, nervousness, excessive sweating, and swelling of tissue behind the eyeball.

-scopy	process of visual examination	laparoscopy _instrumental viewing of the abdomen_ Small incisions are made near the navel, and tubes are inserted into the abdomen for viewing organs and doing procedures such as tying off the fallopian tubes. See Figure 1–7.
		arthroscopy _instru viewing of joints_ See Figure 1–8.
-sis	state of	prognosis _prediction of outcome_
-tomy	process of cutting, incision	neurotomy _process of cutting into the nerves_

Figure 1–7
Laparoscopy.

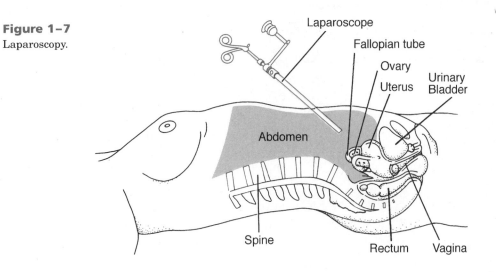

- Laparoscope
- Fallopian tube
- Ovary
- Uterus
- Urinary Bladder
- Abdomen
- Spine
- Rectum
- Vagina

Figure 1–8
Arthroscopy of the knee.

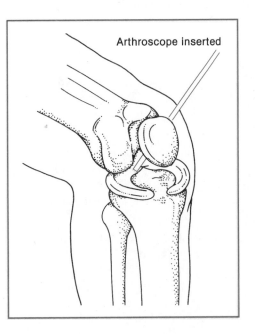

Arthroscope inserted

PREFIXES

Prefix	Meaning	Medical Term	Meaning
a-, an-	no, not	anemia _no blood condition_ Literally, *anemia* means a condition of "no blood." Actually, it is a decrease in numbers of red blood cells or a decreased ability to carry oxygen because of less hemoglobin, a protein that helps carry oxygen in red blood cells.	
aut-	self	autopsy _____ Viewing and examination of a dead body with one's own (self) eyes.	
dia-	complete, through	diagnosis _complete knowledge_	
dys-	bad, painful, difficult, abnormal	dysentery _painful small intestine_ The suffix "y" means condition or process.	
endo-	within	endocrine glands _pertaining to secrete_ CRIN/O means "to secrete" (to form and give off). Examples of endocrine glands are the thyroid gland, pituitary gland, adrenal glands, ovaries, and testes. All these glands secrete hormones *into* the bloodstream.	
exo-	outside	exocrine glands _____ Examples of exocrine glands are sweat, tear, and mammary (breast) glands that secrete substances to the *outside* of the body.	
hyper-	excessive, more than normal	hyperglycemia _excessive blood sugar_ GLYC/O means "sugar." Hyperglycemia is also known as diabetes mellitus. *Mellitus* means "sweet."	
hypo-	below, less than normal	hypodermic _pertaining to below the skin_	

pro-	before
re-	back
retro-	behind
sub-	under, below
trans-	across, through

hypoglycemia _low blood sugar condition_

prognosis _state of knowledge before_

resection _cut out an organ_
-SECTION means "to cut into an organ" but resection means "to cut an organ out in the sense of cutting back or away." The Latin *resectio* means "a trimming or pruning."

retrogastric _pertaining to behind stomach_

subhepatic _pertaining to below the liver_

transurethral _across the urethra_
The urethra is the tube that leads from the urinary bladder to the outside of the body. See Figure 1–2.

III. Exercises

These exercises give you practice writing and understanding the terms presented in Section II. An important part of the learning process involves *checking* your answers with the **answer key** given directly after each exercise. The answers are printed close to the questions so that you can easily check your responses. If you can't answer a question, then *please* look at the answer key and *copy* the correct answer. You may want to photocopy some of the exercises before you complete them so that you can practice doing them many times.

A.   *Using slashes, divide the following terms into their component parts and give the meaning for the whole term:*

1.   adenoma _gland tumor_

2.   arthritis _infl joint_

3.   enteric _pertaining to small intest_

4. encephalitis _inflammation of the brain_

5. dermatosis _abnormal skin condition_

6. oncologist _specialist in tumors_

7. arthroscope _instrument process of viewing a joint_

8. cerebral _pertaining to the brain_

9. cardiology _study of the heart_

10. transhepatic _pertaining to across or thru the liver_

11. cephalic _pertaining to the head_

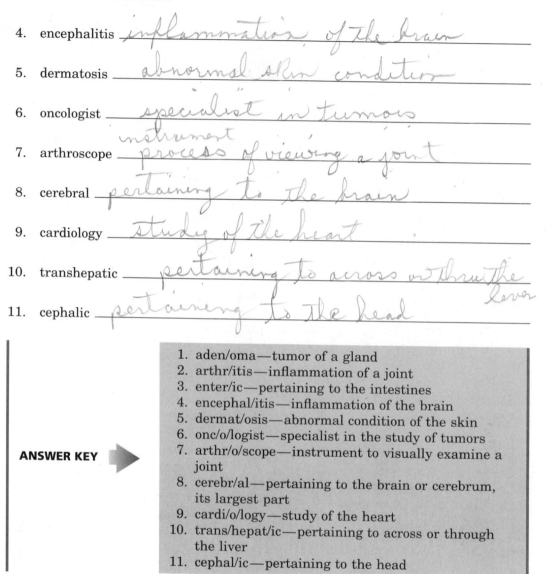

ANSWER KEY

1. aden/oma—tumor of a gland
2. arthr/itis—inflammation of a joint
3. enter/ic—pertaining to the intestines
4. encephal/itis—inflammation of the brain
5. dermat/osis—abnormal condition of the skin
6. onc/o/logist—specialist in the study of tumors
7. arthr/o/scope—instrument to visually examine a joint
8. cerebr/al—pertaining to the brain or cerebrum, its largest part
9. cardi/o/logy—study of the heart
10. trans/hepat/ic—pertaining to across or through the liver
11. cephal/ic—pertaining to the head

B.   *Complete the following medical terms:*

1. _____ gastric   pertaining to under the stomach

2. gastr_____   pain in the stomach

3. gastr_____   inflammation of the stomach

4. _____ gastric   pertaining to across the stomach

5. gastr_____   process of visually examining the stomach

6. _____ gastric   pertaining to behind the stomach

7. gastr_____   instrument to visually examine the stomach

8. gastr_____   study of the stomach and intestines

9. gastr_____   excision (removal) of the stomach

10. gastr_____   incision (to cut into) the stomach

ANSWER KEY

1. subgastric   6. retrogastric
2. gastralgia   7. gastroscope
3. gastritis   8. gastroenterology
4. transgastric   9. gastrectomy
5. gastroscopy   10. gastrotomy

C.   *What part of the body do the following medical terms refer to?*

1. adenoma _____

2. enteritis _____

3. arthrosis _____

4. cerebrovascular accident _____
   (VASCULAR means "pertaining to blood vessels"; a cerebrovascular accident
   is also known as a *stroke*, or *CVA*)

5. dermatitis _____

6. encephalitis _____

7. renal _____

8. osteitis _____

9. nephritis _____

10. electroencephalogram _____

11. rhinitis _____

12. laparotomy _____

13. ophthalmology _____

14. hepatoma _____

ANSWER KEY ➤

1. gland	8. bone
2. intestines (usually small intestine)	9. kidney
3. joint	10. brain
4. brain (cerebrum)	11. nose
5. skin	12. abdomen
6. brain	13. eye
7. kidney	14. liver

D. Divide the following terms into component parts and give their meanings:

1. nephrectomy _____

2. neuritis _____

3. oncology ————————————————————————

4. gastralgia ————————————————————————

5. hepatitis ————————————————————————

6. endocrinology ————————————————————————
   Endocrine glands produce hormones; examples are the thyroid gland in the
   neck, the pituitary gland at the base of the brain, the ovaries in the female,
   and the testes in the male.

7. osteoarthritis ————————————————————————

8. psychology ————————————————————————

9. dermatosis ————————————————————————

10. gynecology ————————————————————————

11. sarcoma ————————————————————————

12. carcinoma ————————————————————————

13. transurethral ————————————————————————

14. ophthalmoscope ————————————————————————

ANSWER KEY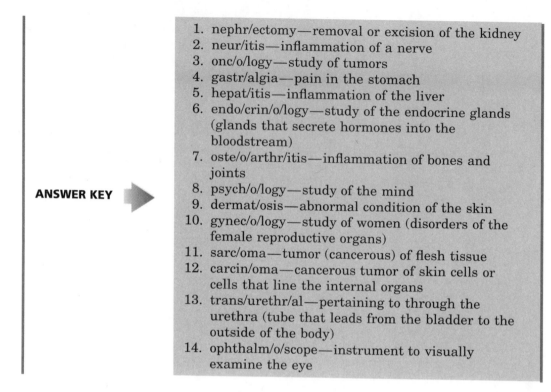

1. nephr/ectomy—removal or excision of the kidney
2. neur/itis—inflammation of a nerve
3. onc/o/logy—study of tumors
4. gastr/algia—pain in the stomach
5. hepat/itis—inflammation of the liver
6. endo/crin/o/logy—study of the endocrine glands (glands that secrete hormones into the bloodstream)
7. oste/o/arthr/itis—inflammation of bones and joints
8. psych/o/logy—study of the mind
9. dermat/osis—abnormal condition of the skin
10. gynec/o/logy—study of women (disorders of the female reproductive organs)
11. sarc/oma—tumor (cancerous) of flesh tissue
12. carcin/oma—cancerous tumor of skin cells or cells that line the internal organs
13. trans/urethr/al—pertaining to through the urethra (tube that leads from the bladder to the outside of the body)
14. ophthalm/o/scope—instrument to visually examine the eye

E.   *Complete the following medical terms:*

1. _____ cyte   A **red** blood cell; these cells carry oxygen to all parts of the body.

2. _____ cyte   A **white** blood cell; these cells help to fight disease.

3. _____ cyte   A **clotting** cell; these cells help your blood to clot and are also called *platelets*.

4. _____ gnosis   A state of **complete** knowledge; what your doctor tells you about your condition after testing and examination.

5. _____ thyroidism   A condition of **excessive** production of hormone from the thyroid gland.

6. _____ thyroidism   A condition of **decreased** production of hormone from the thyroid gland.

7. leuk _____   A **blood condition** of too many white blood cells; the cells are cancerous.

8. _____ logy   Study of **nerves** and nervous disorders.

9. _____ oma   Tumor of the **liver**.

10. _____ logy   Study of **disease**.

ANSWER KEY

1. erythrocyte
2. leukocyte
3. thrombocyte
4. diagnosis
5. hyperthyroidism
6. hypothyroidism
7. leukemia
8. neurology
9. hepatoma
10. pathology

F.   *Identify the suffix in each of the following, and give the meaning of the entire term:*

1. osteotomy _____

2. rhinitis _____

3. neuralgia _____

4. nephrosis _____

5. adenectomy _____

6. cerebral _____

7.   arthrogram _____

8.   laparoscopy _____

9.   laparotomy _____

10.   hepatitis _____

11.   cephalalgia _____

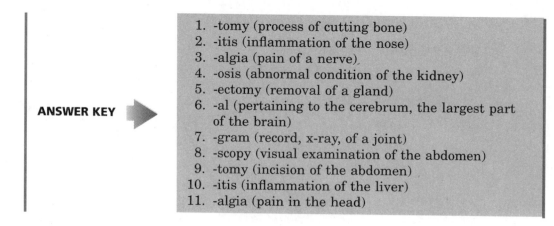

ANSWER KEY

1. -tomy (process of cutting bone)
2. -itis (inflammation of the nose)
3. -algia (pain of a nerve)
4. -osis (abnormal condition of the kidney)
5. -ectomy (removal of a gland)
6. -al (pertaining to the cerebrum, the largest part of the brain)
7. -gram (record, x-ray, of a joint)
8. -scopy (visual examination of the abdomen)
9. -tomy (incision of the abdomen)
10. -itis (inflammation of the liver)
11. -algia (pain in the head)

G.   Give the meaning for the underlined term in each of the following sentences:

1.   An <u>oncologist</u> treats patients who have sarcomas and carcinomas. _____

_____

2.   After explaining Mr. Green's diagnosis to him and outlining the plan of

treatment, Dr. Jones' <u>prognosis</u> was hopeful. _____

_____

3. Seventy-five-year-old Ms. Stein has constant pain in her knees and hips. Her doctor tells her that she has degeneration of her joints and recommends that she take aspirin and other drugs to reduce discomfort from her

   osteoarthritis. _____

4. Thrombosis is a serious condition that can lead to blockage of blood vessels. If the blockage stops blood from reaching body cells, those cells die because

   they are deprived of the food and oxygen that is carried by the blood. _____

   _____

5. A pathologist is the medical doctor who specializes in examining biopsy

   samples and performing autopsies. _____

6. Hyperglycemia can result from a lack of insulin (hormone) secretion from the pancreas (an endocrine gland near the stomach). Without insulin, sugar

   remains in the blood and cannot enter body cells. _____

   _____

7. A patient with a psychosis loses touch with the real world and displays

   abnormal behavior. _____

8. A doctor uses a cystoscope to perform cystoscopy. _____

   _____

9. A <u>laparotomy</u> may be necessary to determine the spread of disease in the

abdomen. _____

10. The doctor used a <u>laparoscope</u> to cut and tie off Ms. Smith's fallopian tubes

so that she couldn't become pregnant. _____

_____

11. Symptoms of <u>hyperthyroidism</u> may include an enlarged thyroid gland,

speeding up of bodily processes, and protruding eyeballs (exophthalmia). _____

_____

12. Mr. Paul had a partial <u>resection</u> of his stomach as treatment for his gastric

adenocarcinoma. _____

13. <u>Leukemia</u> is diagnosed by looking at a blood sample or taking a bone marrow

biopsy. _____

14. A <u>transurethral</u> resection of the prostate gland is a treatment for
    overdevelopment of that gland, which is located below the bladder in

males. _____

15. When Sally returned from her trip to Mexico, she experienced abdominal pain, fever, and severe diarrhea. Her doctor told her she was suffering from

dysentery. ────────────────────────────────────

16. The cerebral blood clot discovered during Mr. Smith's <u>autopsy</u>, confirmed his

doctor's diagnosis of CVA. ────────────────────────────

──

ANSWER KEY ➤

1. specialist in the study of tumors
2. prediction about the outcome of treatment (literally, "before knowledge")
3. inflammation of bones and joints
4. abnormal condition of clotting or clot formation
5. specialist in the study of disease
6. blood condition of too much sugar
7. abnormal condition of the mind
8. process of visual examination of the urinary bladder
9. incision of the abdomen
10. instrument to visually examine the abdomen
11. condition of too much thyroid hormone
12. removal, excision
13. cancerous condition of white blood cells
14. across (through) the urethra
15. painful intestines
16. examination of a dead body

H.   *Circle the term that best completes the meaning of the sentences in the following medical vignettes:*

1.   Selma ate a spicy meal at an Indian restaurant. Later that night she experienced (**osteoarthritis, dermatitis, gastroenteritis**). Fortunately, the cramping and diarrhea subsided by morning.

2.   Christina was feeling very sluggish, both physically and mentally. Her hair seemed coarse, she had noticed weight gain in the past weeks, and she had hot and cold intolerance, never really feeling comfortable. Her internist referred her to a specialist, a(an) (**gynecologist, endocrinologist, pathologist**). The physician did a blood test which revealed low levels of a hormone from a gland in her neck. The diagnosis of (**hypothyroidism, hyperthyroidism, psychosis**) was thus made and proper treatment prescribed.

3.   Dr. Fischer examined the lump in Bruno's thigh. A special imaging technique using magnetic waves and radio signals (an MRI scan) revealed a suspicious mass in soft connective tissue (**hematoma, carcinoma, sarcoma**). The doctor then suggested a(an) (**prognosis, biopsy, autopsy**) to determine if the mass was malignant.

4.   On her seventh birthday, Susie fell down during her birthday party. Her mother noticed bruises on Susie's knees and elbows that seemed to come up "over night." Her pediatrician ordered a blood test that demonstrated lowered thrombocyte count and an elevated (**leukocyte, erythrocyte, platelet**) count at 30,000 cells. Susie was referred to a(an) (**dermatologist, nephrologist, oncologist**), who made a diagnosis of acute (**hepatitis, anemia, leukemia**).

5.   When Mr. Saluto collapsed and died while eating dinner, the family requested a(an) (**laparotomy, gastroscopy, autopsy**) to determine the cause of death. The (**hematologist, pathologist, gastroenterologist**) discovered that Mr. Saluto died of a (**cardiovascular accident, dysentery, cerebrovascular accident**), otherwise known as a stroke.

ANSWER KEY ➡

1. gastroenteritis
2. endocrinologist, hypothyroidism
3. sarcoma, biopsy
4. leukocyte, oncologist, leukemia
5. autopsy, pathologist, cerebrovascular accident

IV. Review

Here's your chance to test your understanding of all the **combining forms**, **suffixes**, and **prefixes** that you have studied in this chapter. Write the meaning of each term in the space provided and *check* your answers with the answer key at the end of each list!

COMBINING FORMS

Combining Form	Meaning	Combining Form	Meaning
1. aden/o	gland	17. gnos/o	knowledge
2. arthr/o	joint	18. gynec/o	woman, female
3. bi/o	life	19. hemat/o	blood
4. carcin/o	cancer	20. hepat/o	liver
5. cardi/o	cancerous heart	21. lapar/o	abdomen
6. cephal/o	head	22. leuk/o	white
7. cerebr/o	brain	23. nephr/o	kidney
8. cyst/o	urine bladder	24. neur/o	neron
9. cyt/o	cell	25. onc/o	tumor
10. dermat/o	skin	26. ophthalm/o	eye
11. electr/o	electricty	27. oste/o	bone
12. encephal/o	brain	28. path/o	disease
13. enter/o	small intestine	29. psych/o	mind
14. erythr/o	red blood cell	30. rhin/o	nose
15. gastr/o	stomach	31. sarc/o	flesh
16. glyc/o	sugar	32. thromb/o	blood clot

SUFFIXES

Suffix	Meaning	Suffix	Meaning
1. -al	pertaining to	10. -opsy	process of viewing
2. -algia	pain	11. -ectomy	excision removal
3. -cyte	cell	12. -emia	blood condition
4. -ic	pertaining to	13. -scope	to visually view with
5. -ism	condition	14. -scopy	process of instrument visual exam
6. -itis	inflammation infection	15. -sis	abnormal condition
7. -logist	specialist in study of	16. -tomy	incision to cut into
8. -logy	study of	17. -osis	abnormal condition
9. -oma	tumor, mass		

PREFIXES

Prefix	Meaning	Prefix	Meaning
1. a-, an-	no not	8. hypo-	below
2. aut-	self	9. pro-	tumor, mass
3. dia-	complete	10. re-	back
4. dys-	bad painful difficult abnormal	11. retro-	behind
5. endo-	within	12. sub-	below
6. exo-	out outside of	13. trans-	across, through
7. hyper-	above, too much		

COMBINING FORMS

1. gland
2. joint
3. life
4. cancerous
5. heart
6. head
7. cerebrum
8. urinary bladder
9. cell
10. skin
11. electricity
12. brain
13. intestines
14. red
15. stomach
16. sugar
17. knowledge
18. woman, female
19. blood
20. liver
21. abdomen
22. white
23. kidney
24. nerve
25. tumor
26. eye
27. bone
28. disease
29. mind
30. nose
31. flesh
32. clot

SUFFIXES

1. pertaining to
2. pain
3. cell
4. pertaining to
5. condition
6. inflammation
7. specialist in the study of
8. study of
9. tumor, mass
10. process of viewing
11. removal
12. blood condition
13. instrument to visually examine
14. process of visual examination
15. condition
16. incision, to cut into
17. abnormal condition

PREFIXES

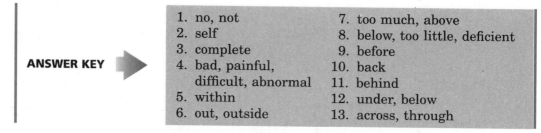

ANSWER KEY

1. no, not
2. self
3. complete
4. bad, painful, difficult, abnormal
5. within
6. out, outside
7. too much, above
8. below, too little, deficient
9. before
10. back
11. behind
12. under, below
13. across, through

V. Pronunciation of Terms

The terms that you have learned in this chapter are presented here with their pronunciations.* The capitalized letters in boldface are the accented syllable. Pronounce each word out loud, then write the meaning in the space provided.

Term	Pronunciation	Meaning
adenitis	ad-eh-**NI**-tis	gland inflammation
adenoma	ad-deh-**NO**-mah	gland tumor
anemia	ah-**NE**-me-ah	no blood condition
arthralgia	ar-**THRAL**-jah	joint pain
arthritis	ar-**THRI**-tis	joint inflammation
arthrogram	**AR**-thro-gram	joint record
arthroscope	**AR**-thro-skop	instrument to view joints
arthroscopy	ar-**THROS**-ko-pe	
autopsy	**AW**-top-se	

*No diacritical (accent) marks are used except ī to indicate the long i in words ending in -CYTE.

biology	bi-**OL**-o-je	study of life
biopsy	**BI**-op-se	process of viewing life
carcinoma	kar-sih-**NO**-mah	cancerous tumor
cardiac	**KAR**-de-ak	pertaining to the heart
cardiology	kar-de-**OL**-o-je	study of the heart
cephalic	seh-**FAL**-ik	pertaining to the brain
cerebral	seh-**RE**-bral	pertaining to the brain
cerebrovascular accident	seh-re-bro-**VAS**-ku-lar **AK**-sih-dent	
cystoscope	**SIS**-to-skop	scope that views the urinary bladder
cystoscopy	sis-**TOS**-ko-pe	
cytology	sī-**TOL**-o-je	study of cell
dermatitis	der-mah-**TI**-tis	skin infection
dermatosis	der-mah-**TO**-sis	abnormal skin condition
diagnosis	di-ag-**NO**-sis	complete knowledge
dysentery	**DIS**-en-te-re	pain of the small intestine
electrocardiogram	e-lek-tro-**KAR**-de-o-gram	record of electricity of the heart
electroencephalogram	e-lek-tro-en-**SEF**-ah-lo-gram	record of the electricity of brain
endocrine glands	**EN**-do-krin glanz	glands that secrete within

Term	Pronunciation	Answer
endocrinology	en-do-kri-**NOL**-o-je	study of glands that secrete within
enteritis	en-ter-**I**-tis	inflammation of small int.
erythrocyte	eh-**RITH**-ro-sīt	red cell
exocrine glands	**EK**-so-krin glanz	glands that excrete outside
gastrectomy	gas-**TREK**-to-me	removal of stomach
gastric	**GAS**-trik	pertaining to the stomach
gastritis	gas-**TRI**-tis	inflammation of stomach
gastroenteritis	gas-tro-en-teh-**RI**-tis	inflammation of study & sml int.
gastroenterology	gas-tro-en-ter-**OL**-o-je	study of stomach sml int. stomach wall
gastroscope	**GAS**-tro-skop	to visually examine instrument
gastroscopy	gas-**TROS**-ko-pe	
gastrotomy	gas-**TROT**-o-me	to cut into stomach
gynecologist	gi-neh-**KOL**-o-jist	female specialist
gynecology	gi-neh-**KOL**-o-je	study of female disorders
hematoma	he-mah-**TO**-mah	a tumor or mass of bl
hepatitis	hep-ah-**TI**-tis	liver inflammation
hepatoma	hep-ah-**TO**-mah	liver tumor
hyperglycemia	hi-per-gli-**SE**-me-ah	above sugar blood condition

hyperthyroidism	hi-per-**THI**-royd-izm	*condition of excessive thy*
hypodermic	hi-po-**DER**-mik	*pertaining to below the skin*
hypoglycemia	hi-po-gli-**SE**-me-ah	*low*
hypothyroidism	hi-po-**THI**-royd-izm	*condition of low thyroid*
laparoscopy	lap-ah-**ROS**-ko-pe	*pou*
laparotomy	lap-ah-**ROT**-o-me	*to cut into abdomen*
leukemia	lu-**KE**-me-ah	*white blood condition*
leukocyte	**LU**-ko-sīt	*white cell*
nephrectomy	neh-**FREK**-to-me	*removal of kidney*
nephrology	neh-**FROL**-o-je	*study of the kidney*
nephrosis	neh-**FRO**-sis	*abnormal condition kidney*
neural	**NU**-ral	*pertaining to the nerves*
neuralgia	nu-**RAL**-je-ah	*pain of the nerves*
neuritis	nu-**RI**-tis	*inflammation of nerves*
neurology	nur-**ROL**-o-je	*study of nerves*
neurotomy	nur-**ROT**-o-me	*to cut into nerves*
oncologist	ong-**KOL**-o-jist	*specialist in tumors*
ophthalmoscope	of-**THAL**-mo-skop	*eye*

osteitis	os-te-**I**-tis	bone inflammation
osteoarthritis	os-te-o-ar-**THRI**-tis	bone joint inflammation
pathologist	pah-**THOL**-o-jist	specialist in disease
platelet	**PLAT**-let	
prognosis	prog-**NO**-sis	predictions of state of knowledge
psychosis	sī-**KO**-sis	abnormal cond of mi
renal	**RE**-nal	pertaining to kidney
resection	re-**SEK**-shun	
retrogastric	reh-tro-**GAS**-trik	pert to back or behind st
rhinitis	ri-**NI**-tis	inflammation of nose
rhinotomy	ri-**NOT**-o-me	to cut into nose
sarcoma	sar-**KO**-mah	tumor or mass of flesh
subgastric	sub-**GAS**-trik	pert to under the stomach
subhepatic	sub-heh-**PAT**-ik	below
thrombocyte	**THROM**-bo-sīt	blood cell
thrombosis	throm-**BO**-sis	blood clot
transgastric	trans-**GAS**-trik	pt across the stomach
transurethral	trans-u-**RE**-thral	pt across the urethra

VI. Practical Applications

Match the **procedure** in Column I with the **diagnosis** that it treats (or helps to diagnose) in Column II. Can you also name the physician who would perform each procedure?

Column I	Column II
Procedure	*Diagnosis*

1. nephrectomy _____ g

2. thyroid gland resection _____ c

3. electroencephalogram _____ e

4. below-knee amputation (resection) _____ f

5. electrocardiogram _____ h

6. gastroscopy _____ d

7. bone marrow biopsy _____ a

8. cystoscopy _____ b

a. leukemia
b. urinary bladder carcinoma
c. adenocarcinoma of an endocrine gland in the neck
d. stomach ulcer
e. seizure disorder (epilepsy)
f. osteogenic sarcoma (bone cancer)
g. renal cell carcinoma
h. heart attack

ANSWER KEY

1. g (urologist)
2. c (head and neck surgeon—an endocrinologist is an internist, not a surgeon)
3. e (neurologist)
4. f (orthopedist)
5. h (cardiologist)
6. d (gastroenterologist)
7. a (oncologist)
8. b (urologist)

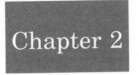

Chapter 2

Organization of the Body

CHAPTER OBJECTIVES

- To name the body systems and their functions
- To identify body cavities and specific organs within them
- To list the divisions of the back
- To identify three planes of the body
- To analyze, pronounce, and spell new terms related to organs and tissues in the body

I. Body Systems

All parts of your body are composed of individual units called **cells**. Muscle, nerve, skin (epithelial), and bone cells are some examples.

Similar cells grouped together are **tissues**. Groups of muscle cells are muscle tissue, and groups of epithelial cells are epithelial tissue.

Collections of different tissues working together are called **organs**. An organ, such as the stomach, has different tissues, such as muscle, epithelial (lining of internal organs and outer layer of skin cells), and nerve that help the organ function.

Groups of organs working together are the **systems** of the body. The digestive system, for example, includes organs such as the mouth, throat, esophagus, stomach, and intestines which bring food into the body and deliver it to the bloodstream.

There are eleven systems of the body, and each plays an important role in the way the body works.

The **circulatory system** (the heart, blood, and blood vessels such as arteries, veins, and capillaries) transports blood throughout the body. The **lymphatic system** also includes lymph vessels and nodes that carry a clear fluid called lymph. Lymph contains white blood cells called lymphocytes that fight against disease and play an important role in immunity.

The **digestive system** brings food into the body and breaks it down so that it can enter the bloodstream. Food that cannot be broken down is then removed from the body at the end of the system.

The **endocrine system**, made up of glands, sends chemical messengers, called hormones, into the blood to act on other glands and organs.

The **female and male reproductive systems** produce the cells that join to form the embryo, fetus, and infant. Male (testis) and female (ovary) sex organs produce hormones as well.

The **musculoskeletal system**, including muscles, bones, joints, and connective tissues, supports the body and allows it to move.

The **nervous system** carries electrical messages to and from the brain and spinal cord.

The **respiratory system** controls breathing, which allows air to enter and leave the body.

The **skin and sense organ system**, including the skin and eyes and ears, receives messages from the environment and sends them to the brain.

The **urinary system** produces urine and sends it out of the body through the kidneys, bladder, and other tubes.

Appendix I, at the back of the book, contains diagrams of each body system along with combining forms for body parts and examples of terminology and pathology. Two glossaries, the Glossary of Medical Terms, page 241, and Glossary of Word Parts, page 273, are alphabetical listings with definitions of terms and meanings of word parts. Use the appendix and glossaries as references during your study and later as you work in the medical field.

II. Body Cavities

Figure 2–1 shows the five body cavities. A body cavity is a space containing
organs. Label Figure 2–1 as you read the following paragraphs.

    The **cranial cavity** (1) is located in the head and is surrounded by the skull
(CRANI/O means "skull"). The brain and other organs, such as the pituitary gland
(an endocrine gland below the brain), are in the cranial cavity.

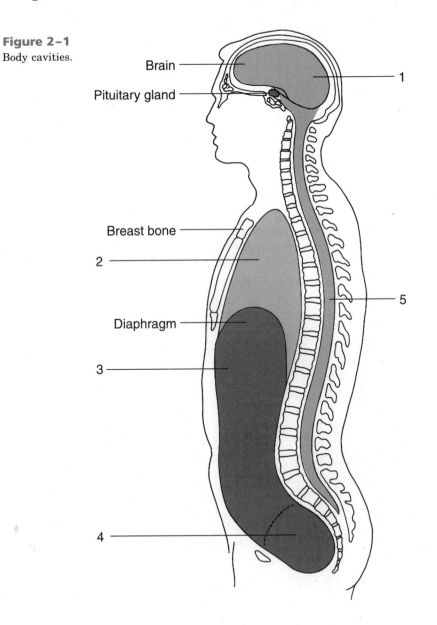

Figure 2–1
Body cavities.

The **thoracic cavity** (2) is the chest cavity (THORAC/O means "chest"), which is surrounded by the breast bone and ribs. The lungs, heart, windpipe (trachea), bronchial tubes (leading from the trachea to the lungs), and other organs are in the thoracic cavity.

Figure 2–2 shows a front view of the thoracic cavity. The lungs are each surrounded by a double membrane known as the **pleura**. The space between the pleura and surrounding each lung is the **pleural cavity**. The large space between the lungs is the **mediastinum**. The heart, esophagus (food tube), trachea, and bronchial tubes are organs within the mediastinum.

Returning to Figure 2–1, the **abdominal cavity** (3) is the space below the thoracic cavity. The **diaphragm** is the muscle that separates the abdominal and thoracic cavities. Organs in the abdomen include the stomach, liver, gallbladder, and small and large intestines.

The organs in the abdomen are covered by a membrane called the **peritoneum** (see Figure 2–3). The peritoneum attaches the abdominal organs to the abdominal muscles and surrounds each organ to hold it in place.

Turn back to Figure 2–1 and locate the **pelvic cavity** (4), below the abdominal cavity. The pelvic cavity is surrounded by the **pelvis** (hip bone). Organs that are located within the pelvic cavity are the urinary bladder, ureters (tubes from the kidneys to the bladder), urethra (tube from the bladder to the outside of the body), rectum and anus, and the uterus (muscular organ that nourishes the developing fetus) in females.

Figure 2–1 also shows the **spinal cavity** (5). This is the space surronded by the **spinal column** (backbones). The **spinal cord** is the nervous tissue within the spinal cavity. Nerves enter and leave the spinal cord carrying messages to and from all parts of the body.

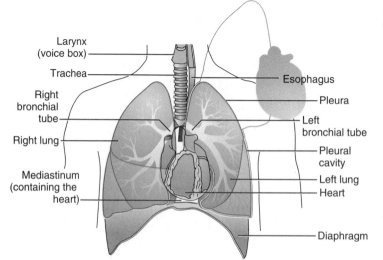

Figure 2–2
Thoracic cavity.

Larynx (voice box)

Trachea

Right bronchial tube

Right lung

Mediastinum (containing the heart)

Esophagus

Pleura

Left bronchial tube

Pleural cavity

Left lung

Heart

Diaphragm

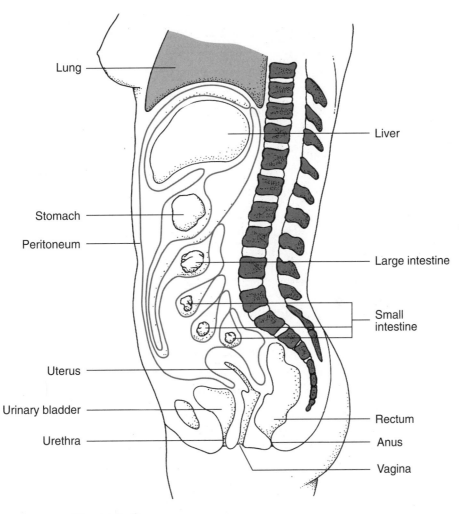

Figure 2–3
The peritoneum as it surrounds the organs in the abdomen.

As a quick review of the terms presented in this section, write the term from the list next to its meaning on the space provided.

Term	Meaning

Abdominal cavity
Cranial cavity
Diaphragm
Mediastinum
Pelvic cavity
Pelvis
Peritoneum
Pleura
Spinal cavity
Thoracic cavity

1. Membrane surrounding the lungs _____

2. Space between the lungs, containing the heart_____

3. Hip bone _____

4. Space containing the liver, gallbladder, and

    stomach; also called the abdomen _____

5. Space within the backbones, containing the spinal

    cord _____

6. Membrane surrounding the organs in the

    abdomen _____

7. Space within the skull, containing the brain_____

8. Space below the abdominal cavity, containing the

    urinary bladder _____

9. Muscle between the thoracic and abdominal

    cavities _____

10. Entire chest cavity, containing the lungs, heart,

    trachea, esophagus, and bronchial tubes _____

III. Divisions of the Back

The **spinal column** is a long row of bones from the neck to the tailbone. Each bone in the spinal column is called a **vertebra** (backbone). Two or more bones are **vertebrae**.

A piece of flexible connective tissue, called a **disk** (also called **disc**), lies between each backbone. The disk, composed of **cartilage**, is a cushion between the bones. If the disk slips, or moves out of its place, it can press on the nerves that enter or leave the spinal cord and cause pain. Figure 2–4 shows a side view of vertebrae and disks.

The divisions of the spinal column are pictured in Figure 2–5. Label them according to the following list:

Division	Bones	Abbreviation
1. **Cervical** (neck) region	7 bones	C1–C7
2. **Thoracic** (chest) region	12 bones	T1–T12
3. **Lumbar** (loin or waist) region	5 bones	L1–L5
4. **Sacral** (sacrum or lower back) region	5 fused bones	S1–S5
5. **Coccygeal** (coccyx or tailbone) region	4 fused bones	

Figure 2–4
Vertebrae and disks.

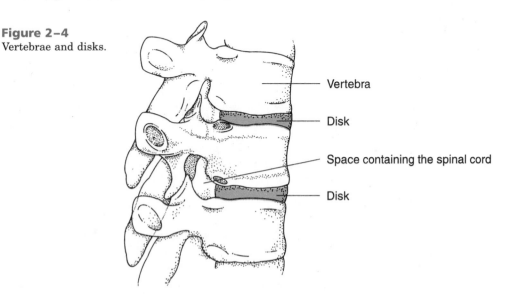

Vertebra

Disk

Space containing the spinal cord

Disk

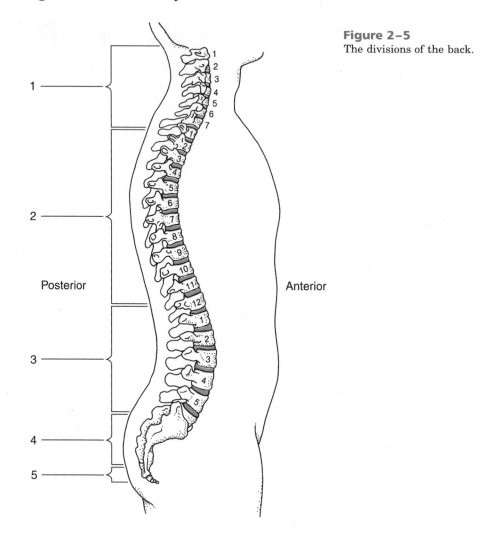

Figure 2–5
The divisions of the back.

Posterior

Anterior

IV. Planes of the Body

A plane is an imaginary flat surface. Organs appear in different relationships to each other according to the plane of the body in which they are viewed.

Figure 2–6 shows three planes of the body. Label them as you read the following descriptions:

1. **Frontal plane** (sometimes called the coronal plane)   An up-and-down plane that divides the body or organ into front (**anterior**) and back (**posterior**) portions. A routine chest x-ray shows the thoracic cavity in the frontal plane. Figure 2–2 shows organs in the frontal plane.

Figure 2–6
Planes of the body.

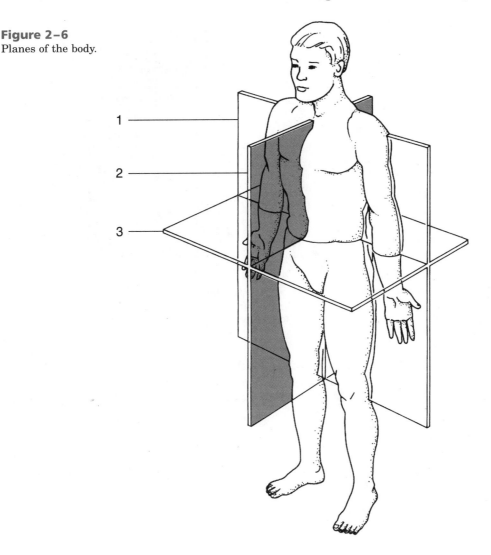

2.   **Sagittal plane**   A plane that divides the body or an organ into a right
                             and left side. Figures 2–1, 2–3, and 2–5 show the body
                             in a sagittal plane, or **lateral** (side) view.

3.   **Transverse plane**   A plane that divides the body or organ into upper and
                             lower portions, as in a **cross-section**. A **CT scan** (CAT
                             scan) is an x-ray picture of the body taken in the
                             transverse plane. Figure 2–7 is a CT scan of the brain.

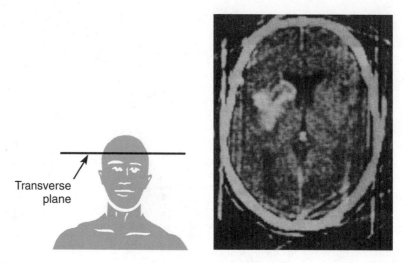

Figure 2–7

CT scan of the brain. Notice the large white region in the brain indicating an area of dead tissue, where a stroke (cerebrovascular accident) has occurred. The figure of the man with the line across his head shows you the transverse plane of the CT scan.

Magnetic resonance imaging (MRI) is another technique of producing images of the body. No x-rays are used, but pictures are made by using magnetic waves. The images from MRI show organs in all three planes (frontal, sagittal, and transverse) of the body. See Figure 2–8.

V. Terminology

Write the meanings of the medical terms on the line provided. Check your answers with the Glossary at the end of the book or with a medical dictionary.

COMBINING FORMS

Combining Form	Meaning	Medical Term	Meaning
abdomin/o	abdomen	abdominal _____	
anter/o	front	anterior _____ The sufix -ior means pertaining to.	

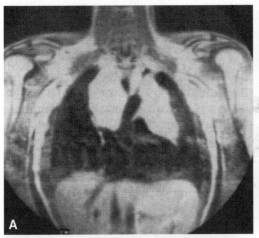

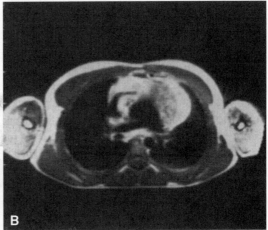

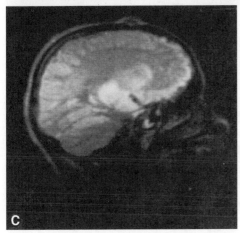

Figure 2–8
Magnetic resonance imaging. *A*, Frontal or coronal view of the chest (white areas indicate tumor). *B*, Transverse view of the chest. *C*, Sagittal (lateral) view of the brain.

bronch/o	bronchial tubes (lead from the windpipe to the lungs)	bronchoscopy _____
cervic/o	*neck* of the body or *neck* (cervix) of the uterus	cervical _____ You must decide from the context of what you are reading whether *cervical* means "pertaining to the neck of the body" or "pertaining to the cervix" (lower portion of the uterus). Figure 2–9 shows the uterus and the cervix.

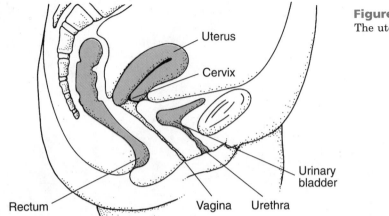

Figure 2–9
The uterus and cervix.

Uterus

Cervix

Urinary
bladder

Rectum

Vagina   Urethra

coccyg/o	coccyx, tailbone	coccygeal _____ -EAL means "pertaining to."
crani/o	skull	craniotomy _____
epitheli/o	skin, surface tissue	epithelial _____ The term *epithelial* was first used to describe the surface (*epi-* means "upon") of the breast nipple (*theli/o* means "nipple"). Currently, it describes cells on the outer layer (surface) of skin and lining internal organs leading to the outside of the body.
esophag/o	esophagus (tube from the throat to the stomach)	esophageal _____
hepat/o	liver	hepatitis _____
lapar/o	abdomen	laparoscopy _____
laryng/o	larynx (voice box)	laryngeal _____ The larynx (**LAR**-inks) is found in the upper part of the trachea.

later/o	side
lumb/o	loin (waist)

laryngectomy _____

lateral _____

lumbar _____
-AR means "pertaining to." A lumbar puncture is the placement of a needle within the membranes in the lumbar region of the spinal cord to withdraw fluid. See Figure 2–10.

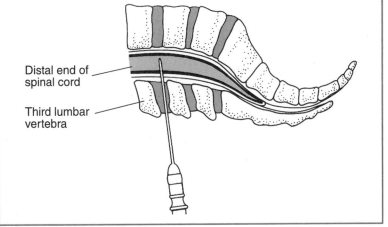

Site of needle puncture

Distal end of spinal cord

Third lumbar vertebra

Figure 2–10

Lumbar puncture. The distal end of the spinal cord is where the spinal cord nerves begin to fan out towards the legs. The lumbar puncture (spinal tap) is made below this area to avoid injuring the spinal cord. Fluid can be injected or withdrawn through the needle.

lymph/o	lymph (clear fluid in tissue spaces and lymph vessels)	lymphocyte _____ Lymphocytes are white blood cells and are important in fighting disease.
mediastin/o	mediastinum (space between the lungs)	mediastinal _____
pelv/o	pelvis (hip bone)	pelvic _____
peritone/o	peritoneum (membrane surrounding the abdomen)	peritoneal _____
pharyng/o	pharynx (throat)	pharyngeal _____ The pharynx (**FAR**-inks) is the common passageway for food from the mouth and air from the nose.
pleur/o	pleura	pleuritis _____
poster/o	back, behind	posterior _____
sacr/o	sacrum (five fused bones in the lower back)	sacral _____
spin/o	spine (backbone)	spinal _____
thorac/o	chest	thoracotomy _____ thoracic _____

trache/o	trachea (windpipe)	tracheotomy _____
vertebr/o	vertebra (backbone)	vertebral _____

VI. Exercises

A. Match the following systems of the body with their functions.

digestive   musculoskeletal   circulatory
respiratory   urinary   endocrine
skin and sense organs   nervous   reproductive

1. Produces urine and sends it out of the body: _____

2. Secretes hormones that are carried by blood to other organs: _____

3. Supports the body and helps it move: _____

4. Takes food into the body and breaks it down: _____

5. Transports food, gases, and other substances through the body: _____

    _____

6. Moves air in and out of the body: _____

7. Produces the cells that unite to form a new baby: _____

8. Receives messages from the environment and sends them to the brain: _____

    _____

9.   Carries electrical messages to and from the brain and spinal cord: _____

_____

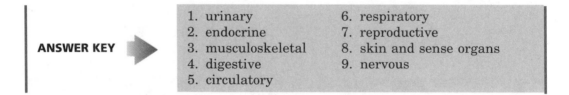

ANSWER KEY

1. urinary   6. respiratory
2. endocrine   7. reproductive
3. musculoskeletal   8. skin and sense organs
4. digestive   9. nervous
5. circulatory

B.   Use the following terms to complete the chart below. Give the name of the cavity and an organ that is contained within the cavity.

spinal   pelvic   cranial
thoracic   abdominal   urinary bladder
stomach   lungs   spinal cord
brain   uterus   heart

	Cavity	Organ
1. Space contained within the hip bone		
2. Space contained within the skull		
3. Space contained within the chest		
4. Space contained within the abdomen		
5. Space contained within the backbones		

ANSWER KEY

1. pelvic (urinary bladder, uterus)
2. cranial (brain)
3. thoracic (lungs, heart)
4. abdominal (stomach)
5. spinal (spinal cord)

C.   *Complete the following sentences using the terms listed below:*

mediastinum   pelvis   vertebra
diaphragm   spinal cord   spinal column
disk   peritoneum   abdomen (abdominal cavity)
                                                  pleura

1.   The hip bone is the _____.

2.   The muscle separating the chest and the abdomen is the _____.

3.   The membrane surrounding the organs in the abdomen is the _____.

4.   The membrane surrounding the lungs is the _____.

5.   The space between the lungs in the chest is the _____.

6.   The space that contains organs such as the stomach, liver, gallbladder, and

     intestines is the _____.

7.   The backbones are the _____.

8.   The nerves running down the back are the _____.

9.   A single backbone is a _____.

10.   A piece of cartilage in between each backbone is a _____.

ANSWER KEY ➤

1. pelvis   6. abdomen or abdominal cavity
2. diaphragm   7. spinal column
3. peritoneum   8. spinal cord
4. pleura   9. vertebra
5. mediastinum   10. disk

D.   *Name the five divisions of the spinal column from the neck to the tailbone.*

1.   C__ __ __ __ __ __ __

2.   T__ __ __ __ __ __ __

3.   L__ __ __ __ __

4.   S__ __ __ __ __

5.   C__ __ __ __ __ __ __ __

ANSWER KEY ➤	1. cervical 3. lumbar 5. coccygeal
	2. thoracic 4. sacral

E.   *Match the following terms with their meanings below.*

transverse plane	CT scan	anterior
frontal plane	sagittal plane	posterior
MRI	cartilage	lateral

1.   Pertaining to the back: _____

2.   Pertaining to the front: _____

3.   A plane that divides the body into an upper and lower part: _____

4.   Pertaining to the side: _____

5.   A picture of the body using magnetic waves; all three planes of the body can

be viewed: _____

6.   A plane that divides the body into right and left parts: _____

7.   Flexible connective tissue found between bones at joints: _____

8. A plane that divides the body into front and back parts: _____

9. Series of x-ray pictures taken in cross-section: _____

ANSWER KEY ➤

1. posterior
2. anterior
3. transverse plane
4. lateral
5. MRI

6. sagittal plane
7. cartilage
8. frontal plane
9. CT scan

F. Give meanings for the following terms.

1. craniotomy _____

2. abdominal _____

3. pelvic _____

4. thoracic _____

5. mediastinal _____

6. epithelial _____

7. tracheotomy _____

8. peritoneal _____

9. hepatitis _____

10. cervical _____

11. lymphocyte _____

12. lateral _____

13.   bronchoscopy _____

14.   diaphragm _____

15.   pleura _____

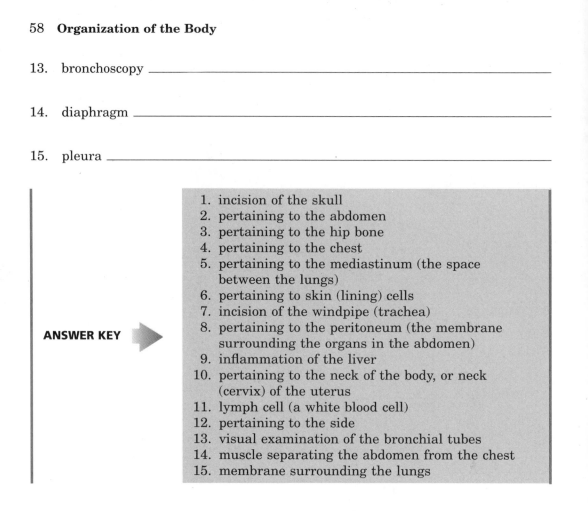

ANSWER KEY ➤

1. incision of the skull
2. pertaining to the abdomen
3. pertaining to the hip bone
4. pertaining to the chest
5. pertaining to the mediastinum (the space between the lungs)
6. pertaining to skin (lining) cells
7. incision of the windpipe (trachea)
8. pertaining to the peritoneum (the membrane surrounding the organs in the abdomen)
9. inflammation of the liver
10. pertaining to the neck of the body, or neck (cervix) of the uterus
11. lymph cell (a white blood cell)
12. pertaining to the side
13. visual examination of the bronchial tubes
14. muscle separating the abdomen from the chest
15. membrane surrounding the lungs

G.   Match the following terms with their meanings below.

pleuritis	pharyngeal	laryngeal	esophageal
epithelial	coccygeal	thoracotomy	lumbar
vertebral	laparoscopy	laparotomy	sacral

1.   Pertaining to the loin (waist) region directly under the thoracic vertebrae: ___

_____

2.   Pertaining to skin or surface cells: _____

3.   Incision of the abdomen: _____

4. Pertaining to the food tube: _____

5. Pertaining to the voice box: _____

6. Inflammation of the membrane surrounding the lungs: _____

7. Pertaining to the throat: _____

8. Pertaining to the sacrum: _____

9. Incision of the chest: _____

10. Pertaining to the tailbone: _____

11. Visual examination of the abdomen: _____

12. Pertaining to backbones: _____

ANSWER KEY

1. lumbar	7. pharyngeal
2. epithelial	8. sacral
3. laparotomy	9. thoracotomy
4. esophageal	10. coccygeal
5. laryngeal	11. laparoscopy
6. pleuritis	12. vertebral

H. *Circle the term that best completes the meaning of the sentences in the following medical vignettes.*

1. After her car accident, Cathy had severe neck pain. An MRI revealed a protruding (**diaphragm, disk, uterus**) at the C7 (**coccyx, ovary, vertebra**). The doctor asked her to wear a (**sacral, cervical, cranial**) collar for several weeks.

2. Mr. Sellar was a heavy smoker all his adult life. He began coughing and losing weight and became very lethargic (tired). His physician suspected a tumor of the (**musculoskeletal, urinary, respiratory**) system. A chest CT demonstrated a (**mediastinal, pharyngeal, spinal**) mass. Dr. Baker performed (**laparoscopy, craniotomy, bronchoscopy**) to biopsy the lesion.

3. Grace had never seen a gynecologist. She had pain in her (**cranial, pelvic, thoracic**) cavity and increasing (**abdominal, vertebral, laryngeal**) girth or size. Dr. Hawk suspected a(an) (**esophageal, ovarian, mediastinal**) tumor, after palpating (examining by touch) a mass.

4. Mr. Cruise worked in the shipyards for several years during World War II. Now, many years later, his doctor encouraged him to stop smoking because of a recent link between asbestos, smoking, and the occurrence of mesothelioma (malignant tumor of cells found in the membrane surrounding the lungs). On routine chest x-ray, there was thickening of the (**esophagus, pleura, trachea**) on both sides of the (**abdominal, spinal, thoracic**) cavity.

5. When Kelly complained of headaches, together with nausea, disturbances of vision, loss of coordination in her movements, weakness, and stiffness on one side of her body, Dr. Brown suspected a tumor of the central (**circulatory, digestive, nervous**) system. Treatment involved a (**thoracotomy, craniotomy, laryngectomy**) to remove the mass in her brain.

ANSWER KEY ➡

1. disk, vertebra, cervical
2. respiratory, mediastinal, bronchoscopy
3. pelvic, abdominal, ovarian
4. pleura, thoracic
5. nervous, craniotomy

VII. Review

Write the meanings of the following combining forms and suffixes in the space provided. Be sure to check your answers with the answer key at the end of each list.

COMBINING FORMS

Combining Form	Meaning	Combining Form	Meaning
1. abdomin/o	_____	14. lymph/o	_____
2. anter/o	_____	15. mediastin/o	_____
3. bronch/o	_____	16. pelv/o	_____
4. cervic/o	_____	17. peritone/o	_____
5. coccyg/o	_____	18. pharyng/o	_____
6. crani/o	_____	19. pleur/o	_____
7. epitheli/o	_____	20. poster/o	_____
8. esophag/o	_____	21. sacr/o	_____
9. hepat/o	_____	22. spin/o	_____
10. lapar/o	_____	23. thorac/o	_____
11. laryng/o	_____	24. trache/o	_____
12. later/o	_____	25. vertebr/o	_____
13. lumb/o	_____		

SUFFIXES

Suffix	Meaning	Suffix	Meaning
1. -ac	_____	7. -ic	_____
2. -al	_____	8. -itis	_____
3. -ar	_____	9. -logy	_____
4. -cyte	_____	10. -oma	_____
5. -eal	_____	11. -scopy	_____
6. -ectomy	_____	12. -tomy	_____

COMBINING FORMS

ANSWER KEY ➤

1. abdomen
2. front
3. bronchial tubes
4. neck
5. tailbone
6. skull
7. skin
8. esophagus
9. liver
10. abdomen
11. voice box
12. side
13. loin, waist region
14. lymph
15. mediastinum
16. hip bone
17. peritoneum
18. throat
19. pleura
20. back, behind
21. sacrum
22. backbone
23. chest
24. windpipe
25. backbone

SUFFIXES

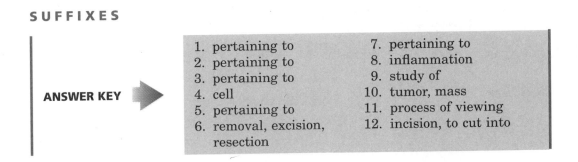

ANSWER KEY

1. pertaining to
2. pertaining to
3. pertaining to
4. cell
5. pertaining to
6. removal, excision, resection
7. pertaining to
8. inflammation
9. study of
10. tumor, mass
11. process of viewing
12. incision, to cut into

VIII. Pronunciation of Terms

The terms that you have learned in this chapter are presented here with their pronunciations.* The capitalized letters in boldface are the accented syllable. Pronounce each word out loud, then write the meaning in the space provided.

Term	Pronunciation	Meaning
abdomen	**AB**-do-men	
abdominal cavity	ab-**DOM**-in-al **KAV**-i-te	
anterior	an-**TE**-re-or	
bronchial tubes	**BRONG**-ke-al tubes	
bronchoscopy	bron-**KOS**-ko-pe	
cartilage	**KAR**-ti-lij	
cervical	**SER**-vi-kal	
circulatory system	**SER**-ku-lah-tor-e **SIS**-tem	
coccygeal	kok-sih-**JE**-al	

*No diacritical (accent) marks are used except ī to indicate the long i in words ending in -CYTE.

coccyx **KOK**-siks _____

cranial cavity **KRA**-ne-al **KAV**-ih-te _____

craniotomy kra-ne-**OT**-o-me _____

diaphragm **DI**-ah-fram _____

digestive system di-**JES**-tiv **SIS**-tem _____

disk (disc) disk _____

endocrine system **EN**-do-krin **SIS**-tem _____

epithelial ep-ih-**THE**-le-al _____

esophageal eh-sof-ah-**JE**-al _____

esophagus eh-**SOF**-ah-gus _____

female reproductive system **FE**-mal re-pro-**DUC**-tive **SIS**-tem _____

frontal plane **FRON**-tal plan _____

hepatitis hep-ah-**TI**-tis _____

laparoscopy lap-ah-**ROS**-ko-pe _____

laparotomy lap-ah-**ROT**-o-me _____

laryngeal lah-rin-**JE**-al _____

laryngectomy lah-rin-**JEK**-to-me _____

larynx **LAR**-inks _____

lateral	**LAT**-er-al _____
lumbar	**LUM**-bar _____
lymphocyte	**LIMF**-o-sīt _____
mediastinal	me-de-ah-**STI**-nal _____
mediastinum	me-de-ah-**STI**-num _____
musculoskeletal system	mus-ku-lo-**SKEL**-e-tal **SIS**-tem _____
nervous system	**NER**-vus **SIS**-tem _____
ovary	**O**-vah-re _____
pelvic cavity	**PEL**-vik **KAV**-ih-te _____
pelvis	**PEL**-vis _____
peritoneal	per-ih-to-**NE**-al _____
peritoneum	per-ih-to-**NE**-um _____
pharyngeal	fah-rin-**JE**-al _____
pharynx	**FAR**-inks _____
pituitary gland	pih-**TU**-ih-tah-re gland _____
pleura	**PLOOR**-ah _lung_
pleuritis	ploo-**RI**-tis _lung inflammation_
posterior	pos-**TER**-e-or _____
respiratory system	**RES**-pir-ah-tor-e **SIS**-tem _____

sacral	**SA**-kral
sacrum	**SA**-krum
sagittal plane	**SAJ**-ih-tal plan
spinal cavity	**SPI**-nal **KAV**-ih-te
spinal column	**SPI**-nal **KOL**-um
spinal cord	**SPI**-nal kord
thoracic cavity	tho-**RAS**-ik **KAV**-ih-te
thoracotomy	tho-rah-**KOT**-o-me
trachea	**TRAY**-ke-ah
tracheotomy	tray-ke-**OT**-o-me
transverse plane	trans-**VERS** plan
ureter	**U**-reh-ter
urethra	u-**RE**-thrah
urinary system	**UR**-in-er-e **SIS**-tem
uterus	**U**-ter-us
vertebra	**VER**-teh-brah
vertebrae	**VER**-teh-bray
vertebral	**VER**-teh-bral

IX. Practical Applications

The following are descriptions of surgical procedures. Can you identify the procedure from its description below? Your choices are:

laparoscopy   craniotomy   thoracotomy
laparotomy   bronchoscopy
laryngectomy   tracheotomy

1. A skin incision is made and muscle is stripped away from the skull. Four or five burr (bur) holes are drilled into the skull. The bone between the holes is cut using a craniotome (bone saw). The bone flap is turned down or completely removed. After the bone flap is secured, the membrane surrounding the brain is incised and the brain is exposed. This procedure is

   called a _____.

2. A major surgical incision is made into the chest for diagnostic or therapeutic purposes. One type of incision is a medial sternotomy (the sternum is the breastbone). A straight incision is made from the upper part of the sternum (suprasternal notch) to the lower end of the sternum (xiphoid process). The sternum must be cut with an electric or air-driven saw. The procedure is done to perform a biopsy, or to locate sources of bleeding or injury. It is often performed to remove all or a portion of the

   lung. This procedure is known as a _____.

3. A needle is inserted below the umbilicus (navel) to infuse carbon dioxide (a gas) into the abdomen, which distends (expands) the abdomen and permits better visualization of the organs. A trocar (sharp-pointed instrument used to puncture the wall of a body cavity) within a cannula (tube) is inserted into an incision under the umbilicus. After it is in place in the abdominal cavity, the trocar is removed and an endoscope is inserted through the cannula. The surgeon can thus visualize the abdominopelvic cavity and

   reproductive organs. This procedure is known as a _____.

4.　A flexible, fiberoptic endoscope is inserted through the mouth, nose, throat, and trachea to assess the tracheobronchial tree for tumors and obstructions, to perform biopsies, and to remove secretions and foreign bodies. This

procedure is called a _____ .

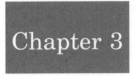

Chapter 3

Suffixes

CHAPTER OBJECTIVES

- To identify and define useful diagnostic and procedural suffixes
- To analyze, spell, and pronounce medical terms that contain diagnostic and procedural suffixes

I. Introduction

This chapter reviews the suffixes that you have learned in the first two chapters and also introduces new suffixes and medical terms. The combining forms used in the chapter are listed below in Section II. Check the list and underline the combining forms that are completely new to you. Refer to this list as you write the meanings of the terms in Section III. Be faithful about completing the Exercises in Section IV, and remember to check your answers! These exercises will help you spell terms correctly and understand their meanings. Test yourself by completing the Review in Section V and Pronunciation of Terms in Section VI.

II. Combining Forms

Combining Form	Meaning
aden/o	gland
amni/o	amnion (sac of fluid surrounding the embryo)
angi/o	vessel (usually a blood vessel)
arteri/o	artery
arthr/o	joint
ather/o	plaque (a yellow, fatty material)
axill/o	armpit (underarm)
bronch/o	bronchial tubes
bronchi/o	bronchial tubes
carcin/o	cancerous
cardi/o	heart
chem/o	drug (or chemical)
cholecyst/o	gallbladder
chron/o	time
col/o	colon (large intestine or bowel)
crani/o	skull
cry/o	cold
cyst/o	urinary bladder; also a sac of fluid or cyst
electr/o	electricity
encephal/o	brain
erythr/o	red
esophag/o	esophagus (tube leading from the throat to the stomach)
hem/o	blood
hemat/o	blood
hepat/o	liver
hyster/o	uterus

inguin/o	groin (the depression between the thigh and the trunk of the body)
isch/o	to hold back
lapar/o	abdomen (abdominal wall)
laryng/o	voice box (larynx)
leuk/o	white
mamm/o	breast (use with -ary, -graphy, -gram, and -plasty)
mast/o	breast (use with -ectomy and -itis)
men/o	menses (menstruation); month
mening/o	meninges (membranes around the brain and spinal cord)
my/o	muscle
myel/o	spinal cord (nervous tissue connected to the brain and located within the spinal column or backbone); in other terms, myel/o means bone marrow (the soft, inner part of bones, where blood cells are made)
necr/o	death (of cells)
nephr/o	kidney (use with all suffixes, except -al and -gram; use ren/o with -al and -gram)
neur/o	nerve
oophor/o	ovary
oste/o	bone
ot/o	ear
pelv/o	pelvic bone (hip bone)
peritone/o	peritoneum (membrane surrounding the organs in the abdominal cavity)
phleb/o	vein
pneumon/o	lung
radi/o	x-rays
ren/o	kidney (use with -al and -gram)
rhin/o	nose
salping/o	fallopian (uterine) tubes
sarc/o	flesh
septic/o	pertaining to infection
thorac/o	chest
tonsill/o	tonsils
trache/o	windpipe; trachea
ur/o	urine or urea (waste material); urinary tract
vascul/o	blood vessel

III. Suffixes and Terminology

Suffixes are divided into two groups, those that describe **diagnoses** and those that describe **procedures**.

DIAGNOSTIC SUFFIXES

These suffixes describe disease conditions or their symptoms. Use the list of combining forms in the previous section to write the meaning of each term. You will find it helpful to check the meanings of the terms with the glossary at the end of book or with a medical dictionary.

Noun Suffix	Meaning	Terminology	Meaning
-algia	pain	arthralgia _____	
		otalgia _____	
		myalgia _____	
		neuralgia _____	
-emia	blood condition	leukemia _____ Increase in numbers of leukocytes; cells are malignant (cancerous).	
		septicemia _____	
		ischemia _____ Figure 3–1 illustrates ischemia of heart muscle caused by blockage of a coronary (heart) artery.	
		uremia _____ Uremia occurs when the kidneys fail to function and urea (waste material) accumulates in the blood.	
-ia	condition, disease	pneumonia _____	

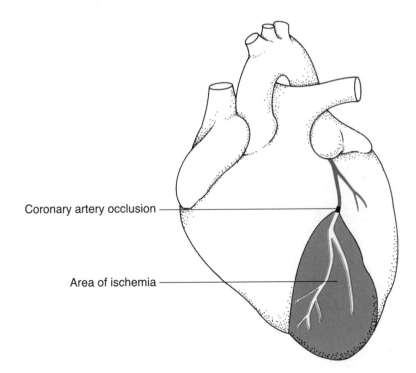

Figure 3-1

Ischemia of heart muscle. Blood is held back from an area of heart muscle by an occlusion (blockage) of a coronary (heart) artery. The muscle then loses its supply of oxygen and food and, if the condition persists, dies. The death of the heart muscle is known as a heart attack (myocardial infarction).

-itis	inflammation	bronchitis _____ See Figure 3-2.
		esophagitis _____
		laryngitis _____
		meningitis _____ The meninges are membranes that surround and protect the brain and spinal cord. See Figure 3-3.
		cystitis _____

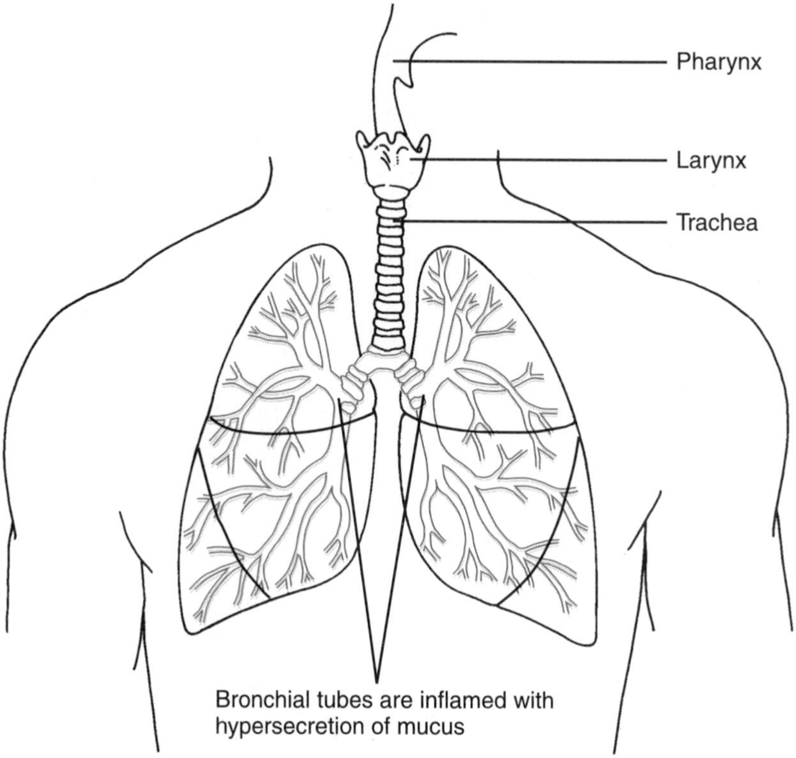

Figure 3–2
Bronchitis.

Pharynx

Larynx

Trachea

Bronchial tubes are inflamed with
hypersecretion of mucus

phlebitis _____

colitis _____
Table 3–1 lists other common inflammatory
conditions with their meanings.

-megaly	enlargement
-osis	condition, abnormal condition

cardiomegaly _____

hepatomegaly _____

nephrosis _____

necrosis _____

erythrocytosis _____
When -OSIS is used with blood cell words it
means "a slight increase in numbers of cells."

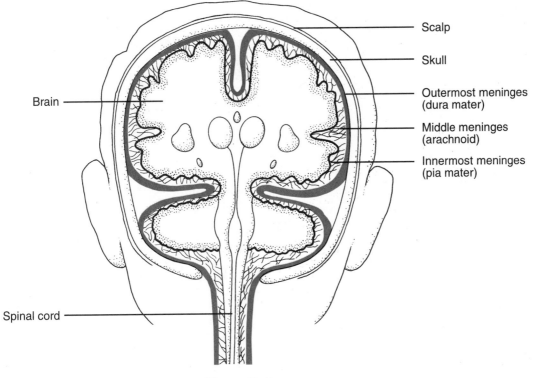

Scalp

Skull

Outermost meninges
(dura mater)

Middle meninges
(arachnoid)

Innermost meninges
(pia mater)

Brain

Spinal cord

Figure 3–3
Meninges (frontal view).

TABLE 3–1.	INFLAMMATIONS
appendicitis	Inflammation of the appendix (hangs from the colon in the lower right abdomen)
bursitis	Inflammation of a small sac of fluid (bursa) near a joint
cellulitis	Inflammation of soft tissue under the skin
dermatitis	Inflammation of the skin
endocarditis	Inflammation of the inner lining of the heart (endocardium)
epiglottitis	Inflammation of the epiglottis (cartilage at the upper part of the windpipe)
gastritis	Inflammation of the stomach
hepatitis	Inflammation of the liver
myositis	Inflammation of muscle
nephritis	Inflammation of the kidney
osteomyelitis	Inflammation of bone and bone marrow
otitis	Inflammation of the ear
pharyngitis	Inflammation of the throat
thrombophlebitis	Inflammation of a vein with formation of clots

-oma	tumor, mass	adenoma _____ This is a benign (non-cancerous) tumor

adenocarcinoma _____
Carcinomas are malignant (cancerous) tumors of epithelial (skin) tissue in the body. Glands and the linings of internal organs are composed of epithelial tissue.

myoma _____
This is a benign tumor.

myosarcoma _____
Sarcomas are cancerous tumors of connective (flesh) tissue. Muscle, bone, cartilage, and fat are examples of connective tissues.

myeloma _____
Myel/o means bone marrow in this term. Also called multiple myeloma, this is a malignant tumor of cells in the bone marrow. See Table 3–2 for names of other malignant tumors that do not contain the combining forms, carcin/o and sarc/o.

hematoma _____
This is not a tumor but a collection of fluid (blood).

-pathy	disease	encephalopathy _____ Pronunciation is en-sef-ah-**LOP**-ah-the.

TABLE 3–2.	CANCEROUS TUMORS, WHOSE NAMES DO NOT CONTAIN THE COMBINING FORMS CARCIN/O AND SARC/O
hepatoma	Malignant tumor of the liver
lymphoma	Malignant tumor of lymph nodes (previously called lymphosarcoma)
melanoma	Malignant tumor of pigmented cells in the skin
mesothelioma	Malignant tumor of pleural cells (membrane surrounding the lungs)
myeloma	Malignant tumor of bone marrow cells
thymoma	Malignant tumor of the thymus gland (located in the mediastinum)

cardiomyopathy _____
Pronunciation is kar-de-o-mi-**OP**-ah-the.

nephropathy _____
Pronunciation is neh-**FROP**-ah-the.

-rrhea	flow, discharge	rhinorrhea _____

menorrhea _____
Normal menstrual flow.

-rrhage or -rrhagia	bursting forth of blood	hemorrhage _____

menorrhagia _____
Excessive bleeding during menstruation.

-sclerosis	hardening	arteriosclerosis _____

Atherosclerosis is the most common type of
arteriosclerosis. A fatty plaque (atheroma)
collects on the lining of arteries. See Figure
3–4.

Figure 3–4
Atherosclerosis (type of arteriosclerosis). A fatty
(cholesterol) material collects in an artery,
narrowing it and eventually blocking the flow of
blood.

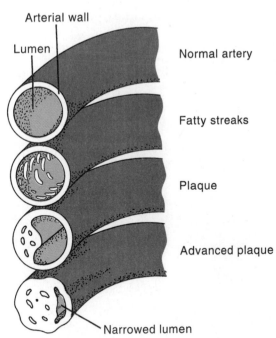

Arterial wall

Lumen

Normal artery

Fatty streaks

Plaque

Advanced plaque

Narrowed lumen

| -uria | condition of urine | hematuria _____
Bleeding into the urinary tract can cause this condition. |

All the following **adjective suffixes** mean "pertaining to" and *describe* a part of the body, process, or condition.

-al or -eal	pertaining to	peritoneal _____
		inguinal _____
		renal _____
		esophageal _____
		myocardial _____ A heart attack is also called a *myocardial infarction* (MI). An infarction is an area of dead tissue caused by ischemia (when blood supply is held back from a part of the body).
-ar	pertaining to	vascular _____ A *cerebrovascular accident* (CVA) is a stroke.
-ary	pertaining to	axillary _____
		mammary _____
-ic	pertaining to	chronic _____ Chronic conditions occur over a long period of time, as opposed to *acute* conditions, which are sharp, sudden, and brief.
		pelvic _____

PROCEDURAL SUFFIXES

The following suffixes describe *procedures* used in patient care.

Suffix	Meaning	Terminology	Meaning
-centesis	surgical puncture to remove fluid	thoracentesis _____ The term is a shortened form of thoracocentesis. See Figure 3–5.	
		amniocentesis _____ See Figure 3–6.	
		arthrocentesis _____	

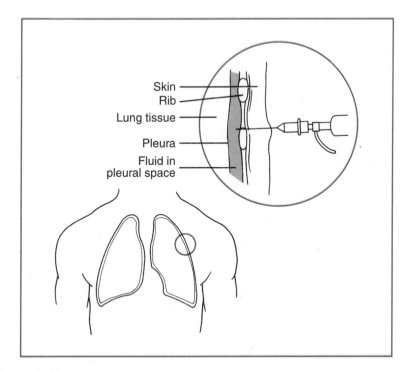

Skin
Rib
Lung tissue
Pleura
Fluid in pleural space

Figure 3–5
Technique of thoracentesis. The needle is advanced only as far as the pleural space.

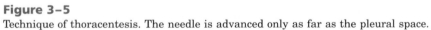

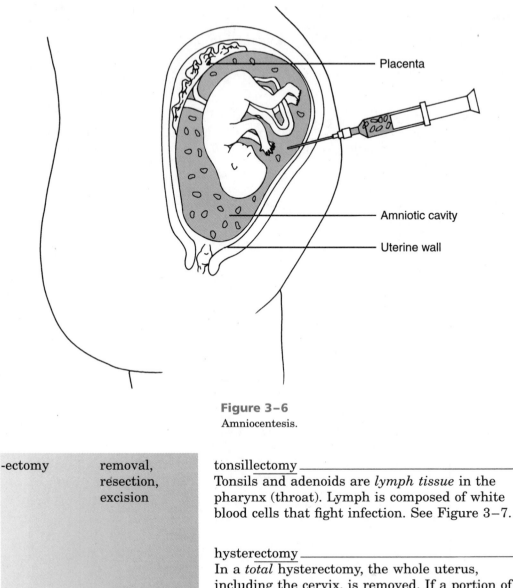

Placenta

Amniotic cavity

Uterine wall

Figure 3–6
Amniocentesis.

| -ectomy | removal, resection, excision | tonsillectomy _____
Tonsils and adenoids are *lymph tissue* in the pharynx (throat). Lymph is composed of white blood cells that fight infection. See Figure 3–7.

hysterectomy _____
In a *total* hysterectomy, the whole uterus, including the cervix, is removed. If a portion of the uterus is not removed, the procedure is termed a *partial* or *subtotal* hysterectomy. See Figure 3–8.

oophorectomy _____

salpingectomy _____ |

Figure 3–7
Tonsils and adenoids. A tonsillectomy and adenoidectomy (T&A) is removal of the tonsils and adenoids.

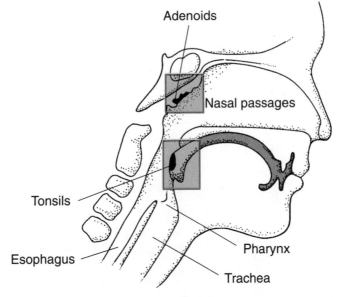

Adenoids

Nasal passages

Tonsils

Esophagus

Pharynx

Trachea

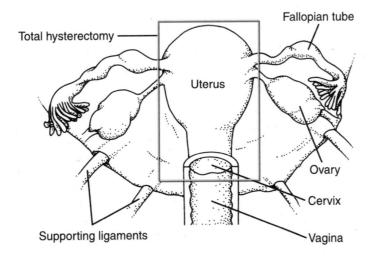

Fallopian tube

Total hysterectomy

Uterus

Ovary

Cervix

Supporting ligaments

Vagina

Figure 3–8
Total hysterectomy. In a total abdominal hysterectomy (TAH), the uterus is removed through the abdomen. A TAH-BSO is a total abdominal hysterectomy with bilateral salpingectomy and oophorectomy.

cholecystectomy _____
See Figure 3–9.

mastectomy _____
Table 3–3 lists additional resection procedures.

-gram   record   myelogram _____
MYEL/O means "spinal cord" in this term. A contrast material is injected into the membranes around the spinal cord (by *lumbar puncture*), and then x-ray pictures are taken of the spinal cord.

mammogram _____
See Figure 3–10.

-graphy   process of   electroencephalography _____
                   recording

angiography _____
Arteriography, phlebography (veins), and lymphangiography are examples of angiography.

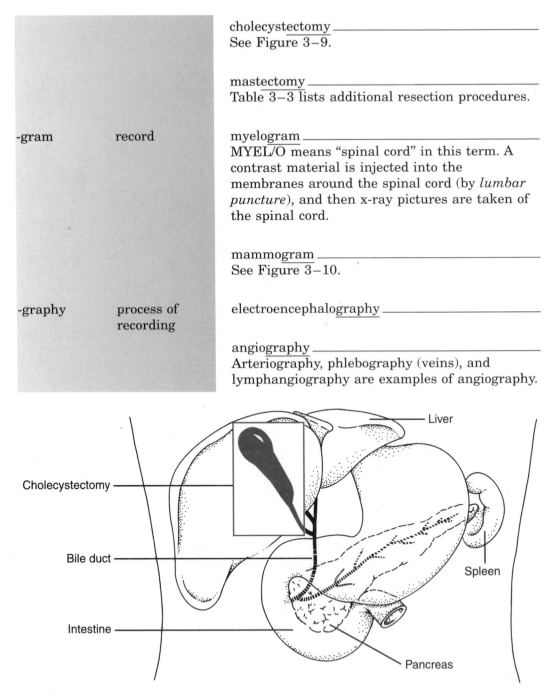

Figure 3–9
Cholecystectomy. The liver is lifted up to show the gallbladder underneath it. The pancreas is a long, thin gland located behind and to the left of the stomach, toward the spleen.

TABLE 3–3.	RESECTIONS
appendectomy	Excision of the appendix
adenectomy	Excision of a gland
adenoidectomy	Excision of the adenoids
colectomy	Excision of the colon
gastrectomy	Excision of the stomach
laminectomy	Excision of a piece of backbone (lamina) to relieve pressure on nerves from a (herniating) disk
myomectomy	Excision of a muscle tumor (commonly a fibroid of the uterus)
pneumonectomy	Excision of lung tissue; total pneumonectomy (an entire lung), or lobectomy (a single lobe)
splenectomy	Excision of the spleen

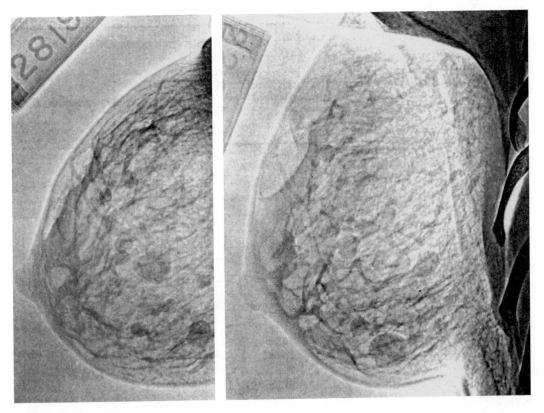

Figure 3–10
Mammograms. Fibrocystic (sacs of fluid and fibrous tissue) masses can be seen in both breasts.

-lysis	separation, breakdown, destruction	

dialysis_____

Hemodialysis is the removal of blood and its passage through (dia- means through or complete) a kidney machine to filter out waste materials, such as *urea*. Another form of dialysis is *peritoneal* dialysis. A special fluid is put into the peritoneum through a tube in the abdomen. The wastes seep into the fluid from the blood during a period of time. The fluid and wastes are then drained from the peritoneum. See Figure 3–11.

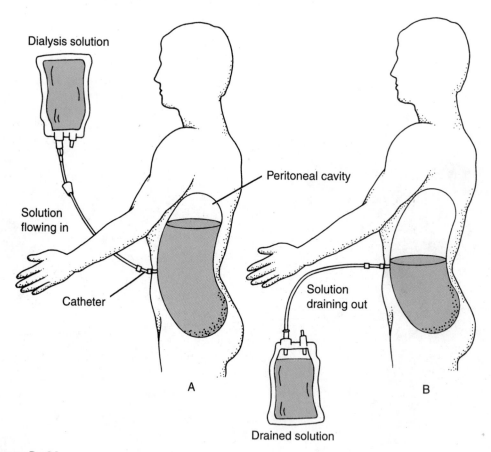

Figure 3–11

Peritoneal dialysis. This procedure (or hemodialysis) is necessary when the kidneys are not functioning to remove waste materials (such as urea) from the blood. Without dialysis or kidney transplantation, uremia can result.

-plasty	surgical repair, or surgical correction	mammo<u>plasty</u> _____ rhino<u>plasty</u> _____ angio<u>plasty</u> _____ Balloon angioplasty is performed on the coronary arteries that surround the heart. A wire with a collapsed balloon is placed in a clogged artery. Opening the balloon widens the vessel, allowing more blood to flow through. See Figure 3–12.
-scopy	process of visual examination	arthro<u>scopy</u> _____ laparo<u>scopy</u> _____
-stomy	opening	colo<u>stomy</u> _____ A -STOMY procedure is the creation of a permanent or semipermanent opening (stoma) from an organ to the outside of the body. See Figure 3–13.

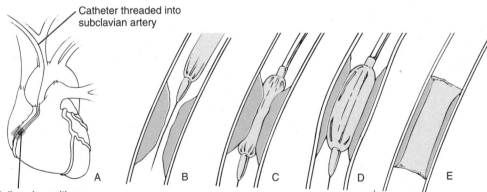

Catheter threaded into subclavian artery

Balloon in position in right coronary artery

A   B   C   D   E

Figure 3–12

Percutaneous transluminal coronary angioplasty (PTCA). (*A*) Balloon-tipped catheter positioned in blocked artery. (*B*) Balloon is centered. (*C*) Balloon expands to (*D*) compress blockage. (*E*) Artery diameter opened. (From Polaski AL and Tatro SE: Luckmann's Core Principles and Practice of Medical Surgical Nursing. Philadelphia, WB Saunders Co, 1996, with permission.)

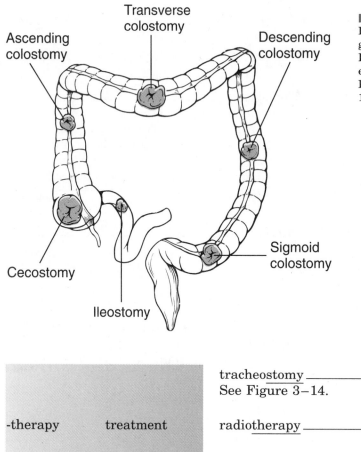

Ascending colostomy

Transverse colostomy

Descending colostomy

Cecostomy

Ileostomy

Sigmoid colostomy

Figure 3–13
Locations of stomas in the gastrointestinal tract. (From Lammon CB, Foote AW, Leli PG et al: Clinical Nursing Skills. Philadelphia, WB Saunders Co, 1995, with permission.)

		tracheostomy _____ See Figure 3–14.
-therapy	treatment	radiotherapy _____
		chemotherapy _____
		cryotherapy _____ Cryoextraction is the application of extremely low temperature for the removal of a cataractous lens of the eye. Cryocautery is burning (cauterization) of tissue by means of application of liquid nitrogen or carbon dioxide snow, or instrument that destroys tissue by freezing.
-tomy	incision, to cut into	craniotomy _____ -TOMY indicates a temporary incision, as opposed to -STOMY, which is a permanent or semipermanent opening.
		laparotomy _____

Figure 3–14
Tracheostomy, with tube in place.

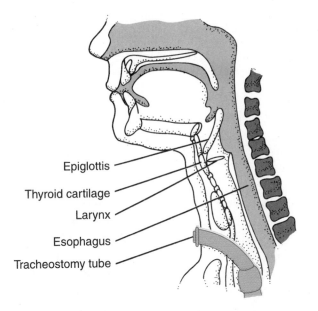

Epiglottis

Thyroid cartilage

Larynx

Esophagus

Tracheostomy tube

IV. Exercises

A. Match the following diagnostic suffixes in Column I with their meanings in Column II.

Column I

Column II

1. -pathy   ____

2. -rrhea   ____

3. -algia   ____

4. -oma   ____

5. -itis   ____

6. -rrhagia   ____

7. -sclerosis   ____

8. -osis   ____

9. -emia   ____

10. -megaly   ____

A. Hardening
B. Discharge, flow
C. Inflammation
D. Blood condition
E. Pain
F. Enlargement
G. Disease condition
H. Tumor, mass
I. Bursting forth of blood
J. Abnormal condition

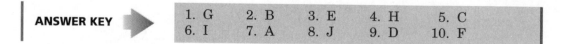
B. *Match the following procedural suffixes in Column I with their meanings in Column II.*

Column I	Column II
1. -tomy ____	A. Removal, resection, excision
	B. Visual examination
2. -scopy ____	C. Process of recording
	D. Opening
3. -therapy ____	E. Record
	F. Separation, breakdown, destruction
4. -stomy ____	G. Treatment
	H. Surgical repair
5. -lysis ____	I. Incision, to cut into
	J. Surgical puncture to remove fluid
6. -centesis ____	
7. -plasty ____	
8. -graphy ____	
9. -ectomy ____	
10. -gram ____	

C. *Select from the following terms to complete the sentences below:*

myalgia	angioplasty	hematuria
septicemia	rhinorrhea	leukemia
thoracentesis	menorrhagia	arteriosclerosis
laryngitis	esophagitis	ischemia

1. Surgical puncture to remove fluid from the chest is —————————

2. Surgical repair of a blood vessel is —————————

3. Muscle pain is —————————

4. Inflammation of the tube leading from the throat to the stomach is —————

5. Holding back blood from an organ or depriving it of blood supply is —————

6. Discharge of mucus from the nose is —————————

7. Blood in the urine is —————————

8. A malignant condition of increase in abnormal white blood cells is —————

9. Hardening of arteries is —————————

10. Excessive discharge of blood during menstruation is —————————

11. Inflammation of the voice box is known as —————————

12. A blood infection is —————————

ANSWER KEY ➡

1. thoracentesis	5. ischemia	9. arteriosclerosis
2. angioplasty	6. rhinorrhea	10. menorrhagia
3. myalgia	7. hematuria	11. laryngitis
4. esophagitis	8. leukemia	12. septicemia

D.   *Underline the suffix and give meanings for the following terms:*

1.   bronchitis _____

2.   encephalopathy _____

3.   pelvic _____

4.   carcinoma _____

5.   chronic _____

6.   otalgia _____

7.   inguinal _____

8.   mastectomy _____

9.   colostomy _____

10.   arthroscopy _____

11.   cardiomegaly _____

12.   hematuria _____

13.   uremia _____

14.   necrosis _____

15.   cryotherapy _____

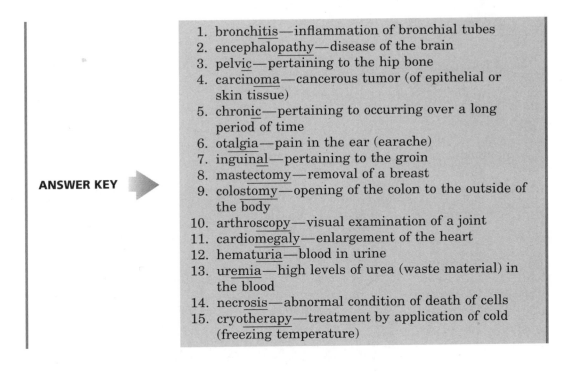

ANSWER KEY

1. bronchitis—inflammation of bronchial tubes
2. encephalopathy—disease of the brain
3. pelvic—pertaining to the hip bone
4. carcinoma—cancerous tumor (of epithelial or skin tissue)
5. chronic—pertaining to occurring over a long period of time
6. otalgia—pain in the ear (earache)
7. inguinal—pertaining to the groin
8. mastectomy—removal of a breast
9. colostomy—opening of the colon to the outside of the body
10. arthroscopy—visual examination of a joint
11. cardiomegaly—enlargement of the heart
12. hematuria—blood in urine
13. uremia—high levels of urea (waste material) in the blood
14. necrosis—abnormal condition of death of cells
15. cryotherapy—treatment by application of cold (freezing temperature)

E. *Name the part of the body described in the following terms and give the meaning of each term:*

1. cholecystectomy _____

2. myalgia _____

3. neuralgia _____

4. nephrosis _____

5. colitis _____

6. myocardial ischemia _____

7. renal _____

8. hysterectomy _____

9.   laparoscopy _____

10.   mammoplasty _____

11.   axillary _____

12.   pneumonia _____

ANSWER KEY ➤

> 1. gallbladder (removal of the gallbladder)
> 2. muscle (muscle pain)
> 3. nerve (nerve pain)
> 4. kidney (abnormal condition of a kidney)
> 5. colon (inflammation of the colon)
> 6. heart muscle (holding back blood to heart muscle)
> 7. kidney (pertaining to the kidney)
> 8. uterus (removal of the uterus)
> 9. abdomen (visual examination of the abdomen)
> 10. breast (surgical repair of the breast)
> 11. armpit (pertaining to the armpit)
> 12. lung (abnormal condition of the lung)

F.   Match the following procedures with their meanings given below:

radiotherapy	colostomy	craniotomy	rhinoplasty
amniocentesis	tracheostomy	electroencephalography	hemodialysis
laparoscopy	chemotherapy	myelogram	laparotomy

1.   Treatment with drugs: _____

2.   Surgical repair of the nose: _____

3.   Separation of waste (urea) from the blood: _____

4.   Opening of the windpipe to the outside of the body: _____

5.   Surgical puncture to remove fluid from the sac around the fetus: _____

6. Incision of the skull: _____

7. Visual (endoscopic) examination of the abdomen: _____

8. Treatment with x-rays: _____

9. Record (x-ray) of the spinal cord: _____

10. Opening of the colon to the outside of the body: _____

11. Process of recording the electricity in the brain: _____

12. Incision of the abdomen (abdominal wall): _____

ANSWER KEY ➡

1. chemotherapy
2. rhinoplasty
3. hemodialysis
4. tracheostomy
5. amniocentesis
6. craniotomy
7. laparoscopy
8. radiotherapy
9. myelogram
10. colostomy
11. electroencephalography
12. laparotomy

G. Match the following abnormal conditions with their descriptions below:

atherosclerosis	hematuria	septicemia	nephrosis
carcinoma	cardiomyopathy	sarcoma	adenoma
myocardial infarction	uremia	hepatomegaly	cerebrovascular accident

1. Malignant tumor of connective tissue: _____

2. Benign tumor of a gland: _____

3. Heart attack (area of dead tissue in heart muscle): _____

4. Hardening of arteries by collection of plaque: _____

5. Stroke (blood vessels in the brain are damaged): _____

6. Disease condition of heart muscle (not a heart attack): _____

7. Abnormal condition of the kidney: _____

8. Blood infection: _____

9. Blood in the urine: _____

10. Excessive urea in the blood: _____

11. Cancerous tumor (of epithelial or surface tissues): _____

12. Enlargement of the liver: _____

ANSWER KEY ➡

1. sarcoma
2. adenoma
3. myocardial infarction
4. atherosclerosis
5. cerebrovascular accident
6. cardiomyopathy
7. nephrosis
8. septicemia
9. hematuria
10. uremia
11. carcinoma
12. hepatomegaly

H. What part of the body is inflamed?

1. neuritis _____

2. arthritis _____

3. salpingitis _____

4. otitis _____

5. hepatitis _____

6. nephritis _____

7. esophagitis _____

8. laryngitis _____

9. encephalitis _____

10. osteitis _____

11. meningitis _____

12. bronchitis _____

13. rhinitis _____

14. peritonitis _____

15. vasculitis _____

16. mastitis _____

17. tonsillitis _____

18. colitis _____

19. pharyngitis _____

20. tracheitis _____

21. phlebitis _____

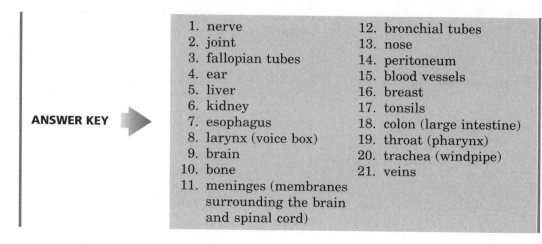

ANSWER KEY

1. nerve
2. joint
3. fallopian tubes
4. ear
5. liver
6. kidney
7. esophagus
8. larynx (voice box)
9. brain
10. bone
11. meninges (membranes surrounding the brain and spinal cord)
12. bronchial tubes
13. nose
14. peritoneum
15. blood vessels
16. breast
17. tonsils
18. colon (large intestine)
19. throat (pharynx)
20. trachea (windpipe)
21. veins

I.   Provide the terms for the following procedures:

1.   Excision of the gallbladder _____

2.   Excision of the appendix _____

3.   Excision of a breast _____

4.   Excision of the uterus _____

5.   Excision of an ovary _____

6.   Excision of the voice box _____

7.   Excision of the kidney _____

8.   Excision of a gland _____

9.   Excision of the large intestine _____

10.   Excision of a fallopian tube _____

11.   Excision of tonsils _____

12. Incision of the skull _____

13. Incision of the abdomen _____

14. Incision of the chest _____

15. Opening of the windpipe to the outside of the body _____

16. Opening of the colon to the outside of the body _____

17. Surgical puncture of the chest _____

18. Surgical puncture of the sac around the fetus _____

ANSWER KEY ➡

1. cholecystectomy
2. appendectomy
3. mastectomy
4. hysterectomy
5. oophorectomy
6. laryngectomy
7. nephrectomy
8. adenectomy
9. colectomy
10. salpingectomy
11. tonsillectomy
12. craniotomy
13. laparotomy
14. thoracotomy
15. tracheostomy
16. colostomy
17. thoracentesis
18. amniocentesis

J. *Select from the following to complete the following definitions:*

adenoma   adenocarcinoma   osteoma   arthropathy
hepatoma   myoma   hematoma   cardiomyopathy
radiotherapy   myosarcoma   encephalopathy   neuropathy

1. Collection (mass) of blood _____

2. Tumor of muscle (benign) _____

3. Treatment using x-rays _____

4. Tumor of a gland (benign) _____

5.   Tumor of bone (benign) _____

6.   Cancerous tumor of glandular tissue _____

7.   Malignant tumor (flesh tissue) of muscle _____

8.   Tumor of the liver _____

9.   Disease of joints _____

10.   Disease of heart muscle _____

11.   Disease of nerves _____

12.   Disease of the brain _____

ANSWER KEY ➡

1. hematoma	7. myosarcoma
2. myoma	8. hepatoma
3. radiotherapy	9. arthropathy
4. adenoma	10. cardiomyopathy
5. osteoma	11. neuropathy
6. adenocarcinoma	12. encephalopathy

K.   *Circle the term that best completes the meaning of the sentences in the following medical vignettes:*

1.   Nora felt a lump in her breast and immediately scheduled an x-ray exam called a(an) (**angiogram, bronchoscopy, mammogram**). The exam showed a stellate (star-shaped) mass that upon biopsy revealed an infiltrating ductal carcinoma. Nora elected to have her breast removed and underwent (**hysterectomy, mastectomy, salpingectomy**), although her physician gave her the option of lumpectomy and (**cryotherapy, thoracotomy, radiotherapy**).

2.   In addition to her surgery, Nora had an (**axillary, inguinal, esophageal**) lymph node dissection to determine if the cancer had spread. Fortunately, this procedure revealed no evidence of metastatic disease in 10 sampled lymph nodes.

3. Sylvia had irregular bleeding in between her periods. She was 50 years old and beginning to undergo menopause. On pelvic exam, Dr. Hawk felt a large, lobulated uterus. Biopsy revealed fibroids, a condition known as (**multiple myeloma, hematoma, leiomyoma, myomas**). The doctor suggested a total abdominal (**gastrectomy, hysterectomy, cholecystectomy**) and bilateral salpingo- (**tonsillectomy, adenoidectomy, oophorectomy**).

4. Victoria had never been comfortable with the bump on her nose. She saw a plastic surgeon who performed (**mammoplasty, rhinoplasty, angioplasty**).

5. Sam was experiencing cramps, diarrhea, and a low-grade fever. He was diagnosed with ulcerative (**colitis, meningitis, laryngitis**) and had several bouts of (**uremia, menorrhagia, septicemia**) because of inflammation and rupture of the bowel wall.

6. Bill was experiencing chest pain every time he climbed a flight of stairs. He went to his doctor who did a(an) (**myelogram, angiogram, dialysis**) and discovered (**adenocarcinoma, nephrosis, atherosclerosis**) in one of his coronary arteries. The doctor recommended a procedure called (**angioplasty, thoracentesis, amniocentesis**). This would prevent further (**otalgia, ischemia, neuralgia**) so that Bill might avoid a (**peritoneal, vascular, myocardial**) infarction or heart attack in the future.

ANSWER KEY

1. mammogram, mastectomy, radiotherapy
2. axillary
3. leiomyoma, hysterectomy, oophorectomy
4. rhinoplasty
5. colitis, septicemia
6. angiogram, atherosclerosis, angioplasty, ischemia, myocardial

V. Review

Write the meanings for the following word parts, and don't forget to check your answers.

SUFFIXES

Suffix	Meaning	Suffix	Meaning
1. -al		15. -megaly	
2. -algia		16. -oma	
3. -ar		17. -osis	
4. -ary		18. -pathy	
5. -centesis		19. -plasty	
6. -eal		20. -rrhage	
7. -ectomy		21. -rrhagia	
8. -emia		22. -rrhea	
9. -gram		23. -sclerosis	
10. -graphy		24. -scopy	
11. -ia		25. -stomy	
12. -ic		26. -therapy	
13. -itis		27. -tomy	
14. -lysis		28. -uria	

COMBINING FORMS

Combining Form	Meaning	Combining Form	Meaning
1. aden/o	_____	17. cyst/o	_____
2. amni/o	_____	18. encephal/o	_____
3. angi/o	_____	19. erythr/o	_____
4. arteri/o	_____	20. esophag/o	_____
5. arthr/o	_____	21. hemat/o	_____
6. ather/o	_____	22. hepat/o	_____
7. axill/o	_____	23. hyster/o	_____
8. bronch/o	_____	24. inguin/o	_____
9. carcin/o	_____	25. isch/o	_____
10. cardi/o	_____	26. lapar/o	_____
11. chem/o	_____	27. laryng/o	_____
12. cholecyst/o	_____	28. leuk/o	_____
13. chron/o	_____	29. mamm/o	_____
14. col/o	_____	30. mast/o	_____
15. crani/o	_____	31. men/o	_____
16. cry/o	_____	32. mening/o	_____

33. my/o _____

34. myel/o _____

35. necr/o _____

36. nephr/o _____

37. neur/o _____

38. oophor/o _____

39. oste/o _____

40. ot/o _____

41. pelv/o _____

42. peritone/o _____

43. phleb/o _____

44. pneumon/o _____

45. radi/o _____

46. ren/o _____

47. rhin/o _____

48. salping/o _____

49. sarc/o _____

50. septic/o _____

51. thorac/o _____

52. tonsill/o _____

53. trache/o _____

54. ur/o _____

55. vascul/o _____

SUFFIXES

1. pertaining to
2. pain
3. pertaining to
4. pertaining to
5. surgical puncture to remove fluid
6. pertaining to
7. removal, resection, excision
8. blood condition
9. record
10. process of recording
11. condition
12. pertaining to
13. inflammation
14. separation, breakdown, destruction
15. enlargement
16. tumor, mass
17. abnormal condition
18. disease condition
19. surgical repair
20. bursting forth of blood
21. bursting forth of blood
22. flow, discharge
23. hardening
24. visual examination
25. opening
26. treatment
27. incision
28. urine condition

COMBINING FORMS

1. gland
2. amnion
3. blood vessel
4. artery
5. joint
6. plaque, collection of fatty material
7. armpit
8. bronchial tubes
9. cancerous
10. heart
11. drug, chemical
12. gallbladder
13. time
14. colon (large intestine)
15. skull
16. cold
17. urinary bladder
18. brain
19. red
20. esophagus
21. blood
22. liver
23. uterus
24. groin
25. to hold back
26. abdomen
27. larynx (voice box)
28. white
29. breast
30. breast
31. menstruation
32. meninges
33. muscle
34. spinal cord or bone marrow
35. death
36. kidney
37. nerve
38. ovary
39. bone
40. ear
41. hip bone
42. peritoneum
43. vein
44. lungs
45. x-rays
46. kidney
47. nose
48. fallopian tube
49. flesh
50. pertaining to infection
51. chest
52. tonsils
53. trachea (windpipe)
54. urine, urinary tract
55. blood vessel

VI. Pronunciation of Terms

The terms that you have learned in this chapter are presented here with their pronunciations. The capitalized letters in boldface are the accented syllable. Pronounce each word out loud, then write the meaning in the space provided.

Term	Pronunciation	Meaning
acute	ah-**KUT**	
adenocarcinoma	ah-deh-no-kar-sih-**NO**-mah	
adenoma	ah-deh-**NO**-mah	
amniocentesis	am-ne-o-sen-**TE**-sis	
angiography	an-je-**OG**-rah-fe	
angioplasty	**AN**-je-o-plas-te	
arteriosclerosis	ar-ter-i-o-skle-**RO**-sis	
arthralgia	ar-**THRAL**-je-ah	
arthropathy	ar-**THROP**-ah-the	
arthroscopy	ar-**THROS**-ko-pe	
atherosclerosis	ah-theh-ro-skle-**RO**-sis	
axillary	**AKS**-ih-lar-e	
bronchitis	brong-**KI**-tis	
carcinoma	kar-sih-**NO**-mah	

cardiomegaly	kar-de-o-**MEG**-ah-le _____
cardiomyopathy	kar-de-o-mi-**OP**-ah-the _____
chemotherapy	ke-mo-**THER**-ah-pe _____
cholecystectomy	ko-le-sis-**TEK**-to-me _____
chronic	**KRON**-ik _____
colitis	ko-**LI**-tis _____
colostomy	ko-**LOS**-to-me _____
craniotomy	kra-ne-**OT**-o-me _____
cystitis	sis-**TI**-tis _____
dialysis	di-**AL**-ih-sis _____
electroencephalography	e-lek-tro-en-sef-ah-**LOG**-rah-fe _____
encephalopathy	en-sef-ah-**LOP**-ah-the _____
erythrocytosis	eh-rith-ro-si-**TO**-sis _____
esophageal	e-sof-ah-**JE**-al _____
esophagitis	e-sof-ah-**JI**-tis _____
hematoma	he-mah-**TO**-mah _____
hematuria	he-mah-**TUR**-e-ah _____
hemorrhage	**HEM**-or-ij _____

hysterectomy	his-teh-**REK**-to-me _____
infarction	in-**FARK**-shun _____
inguinal	**ING**-gwi-nal _____
ischemia	is-**KE**-me-ah _____
laparoscopy	lap-ah-**ROS**-ko-pe _____
laparotomy	lap-ah-**ROT**-o-me _____
laryngitis	lah-rin-**JI**-tis _____
leukemia	lu-**KE**-me-ah _____
mammogram	**MAM**-o-gram _____
mammography	ma-**MOG**-rah-fe _____
mammoplasty	**MAM**-o-plas-te _____
mastectomy	mas-**TEK**-to-me _____
meningitis	men-in-**JI**-tis _____
menorrhagia	men-or-**RA**-jah/men-or-**RA**-je-ah _____
menorrhea	men-o-**RE**-ah _____
myalgia	mi-**AL**-je-ah _____
myelogram	**MI**-eh-lo-gram _____
myeloma	mi-eh-**LO**-mah _____

myocardial	mi-o-**KAR**-de-al _____
myoma	mi-**O**-mah _____
myosarcoma	mi-o-sar-**KO**-mah _____
necrosis	neh-**KRO**-sis _____
nephrosis	neh-**FRO**-sis _____
neuralgia	nu-**RAL**-je-ah _____
oophorectomy	o-of-o-**REK**-to-me/oo-for-**REK**-to-me _____
otalgia	o-**TAL**-je-ah _____
pelvic	**PEL**-vik _____
peritoneal	per-ih-to-**NE**-al _____
phlebitis	fle-**BI**-tis _____
radiotherapy	ra-de-o-**THER**-ah-pe _____
renal	**RE**-nal _____
rhinoplasty	**RI**-no-plas-te _____
rhinorrhea	ri-no-**RE**-ah _____
salpingectomy	sal-ping-**JEK**-to-me _____
septicemia	sep-ti-**SE**-me-ah _____
thoracentesis	tho-rah-sen-**TE**-sis _____

tonsillectomy	ton-si-**LEK**-to-me _____
tracheostomy	tra-ke-**OS**-to-me _____
uremia	u-**RE**-me-ah _____
vascular	**VAS**-ku-lar _____

VII. Practical Applications

A. *Match the procedure in Column I with an abnormal condition it treats or diagnoses in Column II:*

Column I	Column II
Procedure	*Abnormal Condition*

1. angioplasty	_____	A. uterine adenocarcinoma
		B. ligament tear of the patella (knee cap)
2. mammoplasty	_____	C. ovarian cyst
		D. blockage of the windpipe
3. cholecystectomy	_____	E. renal failure
		F. absence of a breast (post-mastectomy)
4. tonsillectomy	_____	G. pleural effusion (collection of fluid)
		H. coronary atherosclerosis
5. dialysis	_____	I. gallbladder calculi (stones)
		J. pharyngeal lymph node enlargement
6. hysterectomy	_____	
7. thoracentesis	_____	
8. oophorectomy	_____	
9. tracheostomy	_____	
10. arthroscopy	_____	

(Continued)

B. **Match the symptom or abnormal condition in Column I with the organ or tissue affected in Column II:**

Column I	Column II
Symptom or Abnormal Condition	*Organ or Tissue*

1. colitis   _____   A. uterus
                                   B. ear
2. phlebitis   _____   C. bone marrow
                                   D. coronary arteries
3. menorrhagia   _____   E. large bowel
                                   F. spinal cord or brain
4. myocardial ischemia _____   G. vein
                                   H. kidney
5. otalgia   _____

6. uremia   _____

7. meningitis   _____

8. leukemia   _____

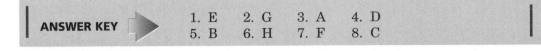

Prefixes

C H A P T E R   O B J E C T I V E S

- To identify and define common prefixes used in medical terms
- To analyze, spell, and pronounce medical terms that contain prefixes

I. Introduction

This chapter includes prefixes that were introduced in Chapter 1 and adds new prefixes as well. The list of Combining Forms and Suffixes in Section II helps you understand the Prefixes and Terminology in Section III. Complete the Exercises in Section IV and the Review in Section V. Don't forget to check your answers! The answers to exercises are placed directly after the questions so that you can use them easily. The Pronunciation of Terms in Section VI is your final review of the terminology in this chapter.

II. Combining Forms and Suffixes

Combining Form	Meaning
abdomin/o	abdomen
an/o	anus (opening of the digestive tract to the outside of the body)
bi/o	life
cardi/o	heart
carp/o	carpals (wrist bones)
cis/o	to cut
cost/o	ribs
crani/o	skull
cutane/o	skin
dur/o	dura mater (outermost meningeal membrane surrounding the brain and spinal cord)
gen/o	to produce, to begin
glyc/o	sugar
hemat/o	blood
later/o	side
men/o	menses (monthly discharge of blood from the lining of the uterus)
nat/i	birth
norm/o	rule, order
oste/o	bone
peritone/o	peritoneum (membrane surrounding the organs in the abdomen)
plas/o	formation, growth, development
ren/o	kidney
scapul/o	scapula (shoulder blade)
son/o	sound

thyroid/o	thyroid gland
top/o	to put, place, position
troph/o	development, nourishment
urethr/o	urethra (tube leading from the bladder to the outside of the body)
uter/o	uterus
ven/o	vein
vertebr/o	vertebra (backbone)

Suffix	Meaning
-al	pertaining to
-ation	process, condition
-cision	process of cutting
-crine	secretion
-emia	blood condition
-gen	to produce
-graphy	process of recording
-ia	condition, process
-ic	pertaining to
-ine	pertaining to
-ism	condition, process
-lapse	to fall, slide
-lysis	loosening, breakdown, separation, destruction
-mission	to send
-mortem	death
-oma	tumor, mass
-ous	pertaining to
-partum	birth
-phagia	to eat, swallow
-phasia	to speak
-plasm	formation
-plegia	paralysis
-pnea	breathing
-rrhea	flow, discharge
-scopy	process of visual examination
-section	to cut
-stasis	to stand, place, stop, control
-tension	pressure
-thesis	to put, place
-tic	pertaining to
-um	structure
-uria	urine condition
-y	process, condition

III. Prefixes and Terminology

Prefix	Meaning	Terminology	Meaning
a-, an-	no, not, without	apnea _____	
		aphasia _____ A stroke on the left side of the brain can produce this condition.	
		atrophy _____ Muscular atrophy can occur because of disuse of the muscle.	
		anemia _____ Anemia is a lower number of red blood cells or a decrease in hemoglobin in the cells. Table 4–1 lists some of the different forms of anemia.	
		amenorrhea _____	
ab-	away from	abnormal _____	
ad-	toward, near	adrenal glands _____ See Figure 4–1.	

TABLE 4–1.	ANEMIAS
aplastic anemia	Bone marrow fails to produce red blood cells (erythrocytes), white blood cells (leukocytes), and clotting cells (platelets).
hemolytic anemia	Red blood cells are destroyed (-lytic), and bone marrow cannot compensate for their loss. This condition can be hereditary or acquired (after infection or chemotherapy) or can occur when the immune system acts against normal red blood cells (autoimmune condition).
iron deficiency anemia	Low or absent iron levels lead to low hemoglobin concentration or deficiency of red blood cells.
pernicious anemia	The mucous membrane of the stomach fails to produce a factor (intrinsic factor) that is necessary for the absorption of vitamin B_{12} and the proper formation of red blood cells.
sickle cell anemia	Erythrocytes assume an abnormal crescent or sickle shape; it is caused by the inheritance of an abnormal type of hemoglobin. The sickle-shaped cells clump together, causing clots that block blood vessels.

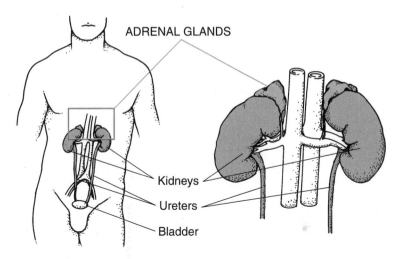

Figure 4–1
Adrenal glands. These two endocrine glands are above each kidney.

ana-	up, apart	analysis _____
		A *urinalysis* (urine + analysis) is a separation of urine to determine its parts.
ante-	before, forward	ante partum _____
		ante mortem _____
anti-	against	antibodies _____
		Antibodies are proteins that are made by white blood cells; literally, they are "bodies" that are "against" foreign substances.
		antigen _____
		Antigens are foreign substances, such as bacteria and viruses. When antigens enter the body, they stimulate white blood cells to produce antibodies that act against the antigens. Think of the ANTI in *antigen* as standing for antibody, so that *antigen* means "to produce (-gen) antibodies."

antibiotic _____
Antibiotics differ from antibodies in that they
are produced *outside* the body by primitive
plants called molds. Examples of antibiotics are
penicillin and erythromycin.

bi-	two, both	bilateral _____
brady-	slow	bradycardia _____
con-	with, together	congenital

congenital
A congenital anomaly is an irregularity
(anomaly) present at birth. Examples are
webbed fingers and toes and heart defects.

dia-	through, complete	diarrhea _____

dialysis _____
-LYSIS means "separation" here.

dys-	bad, painful, difficult, abnormal	dyspnea _____

dysphagia _____

dysplasia _____

dysmenorrhea _____

dysuria _____

ec-	out, outside	ectopic pregnancy _____

Figure 4–2 shows possible sites of ectopic
pregnancies. Figure 4–3 indicates uterine levels
in a normal pregnancy.

endo-	within, in, inner	endoscopy _____

Table 4–2 lists examples of endoscopies.

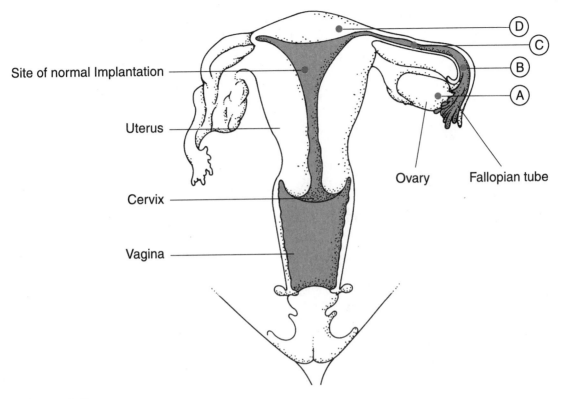

Site of normal Implantation

Uterus

Cervix

Vagina

Ovary   Fallopian tube

Figure 4–2
Ectopic pregnancy. A, B, C, and D are ectopic sites. The fallopian tube is the most common site for ectopic pregnancies (95%), but they can also occur on the ovary or on the surface of the peritoneum. Normal implantation takes place on the inner lining (endometrium) of the uterus.

		endocrine glands _____ The adrenal glands are endocrine glands.
epi-	above, upon	epidural hematoma _____ Figure 4–4 illustrates epidural and subdural hematomas.
		epidermis _____ The three layers of the skin, from outermost to innermost, are the epidermis, dermis, and subcutaneous layer. Check *Appendix I* (Skin and Sense Organs) for a diagram of the skin.
ex-	out	excision _____

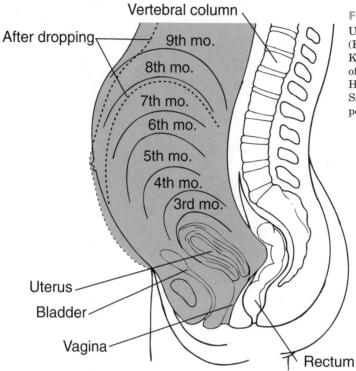

After dropping

Vertebral column

9th mo.
8th mo.
7th mo.
6th mo.
5th mo.
4th mo.
3rd mo.

Uterus

Bladder

Vagina

Rectum

Figure 4–3

Uterine levels in pregnancy. (From O'Toole M [ed]: Miller-Keane Encyclopedia & Dictionary of Medicine, Nursing, & Allied Health, 6th ed. Philadelphia, WB Saunders Co, 1996, with permission.)

TABLE 4–2.	ENDOSCOPIES
arthroscopy	Visual examination of a joint
bronchoscopy	Visual examination of the bronchial tubes
colonoscopy	Visual examination of the colon (large intestine)
cystoscopy	Visual examination of the urinary bladder
esophagoscopy	Visual examination of the esophagus
gastroscopy	Visual examination of the stomach
hysteroscopy	Visual examination of the uterus
laparoscopy	Visual examination of the abdomen
laryngoscopy	Visual examination of the larynx (voice box)
mediastinoscopy	Visual examination of the mediastinum
proctosigmoidoscopy	Visual examination of the rectum and sigmoid colon
sigmoidoscopy	Visual examination of the sigmoid colon (lower, S-shaped part of the large intestine)

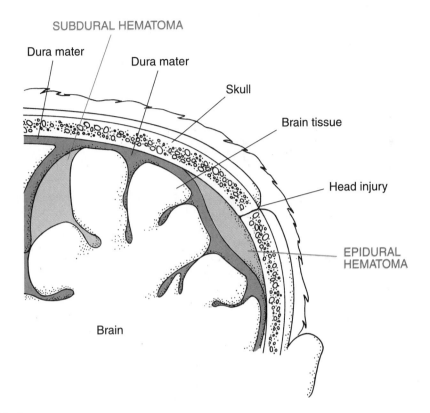

Figure 4–4
Epidural and subdural hematomas. The dura mater is the outermost of the three meninges (membranes) around the brain and spinal cord.

extra-	outside of	extrahepatic _____
hemi-	half	hemigastrectomy _____
		hemiplegia _____
		One side of the body is paralyzed; usually caused by a cerebral vascular accident or a brain lesion, such as a tumor. The paralysis occurs on the side opposite the brain disorder.
hyper-	excessive, above	hyperthyroidism _____
		Figure 4–5 shows the position of the thyroid gland in the neck.

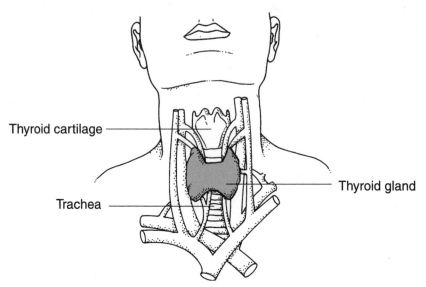

Figure 4–5

Thyroid gland, located in front of the trachea in the neck. The thyroid gland produces too much hormone in hyperthyroidism (Graves disease).

hypertrophy _____
Cells increase in size, not in number. The opposite of hypertrophy is *atrophy* (cells shrink in size).

hypertension _____
Risk factors that contribute to high blood pressure are increasing age, smoking, obesity, heredity, and a stressful life style.

hyperglycemia _____
Also known as diabetes mellitus. *Mellitus* means "sweet." Insulin is either not secreted or improperly utilized so that sugar accumulates in the bloodstream and "spills over" into the urine.

hypo-   below, deficient

hypoglycemia _____
Overproduction of insulin or an overdose (from outside the body—exogenously) of insulin can lead to hypoglycemia, as glucose is removed from the blood at an increased rate.

in-	in, into	incision _____
inter-	between	intervertebral _____
intra-	within	intrauterine _____
		intravenous _____

mal-   bad   malignant
-IGNANT comes from the Latin *ignis* meaning a "fire." A malignant tumor is a cancerous growth. A *benign* tumor (*ben* means "good") is a non-cancerous growth.

meta-   change, beyond   metastasis _____
This term literally means a change of place (-stasis). It is the spread of a cancerous tumor from its original place to a secondary location in the body.

metacarpals _____
The carpal bones are the wrist bones, and the metacarpals are the hand bones, which are "beyond the wrist." See the x-ray picture of the hand in Figure 4–6.

neo-   new   neoplasm _____

neoplastic _____

neonatal _____

para-   beside, near, along the side of   parathyroid glands _____
Figure 4–7 shows the position of the parathyroid glands on the back side of the thyroid gland. The parathyroid glands are endocrine glands that regulate the amount of calcium in bones and in the blood.

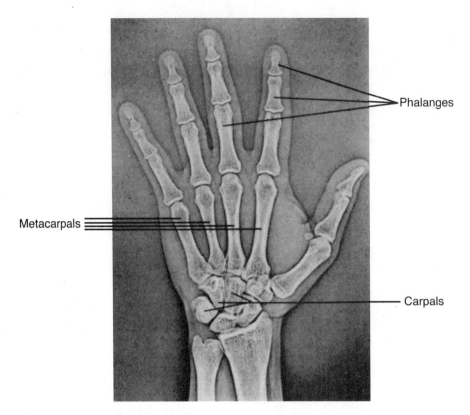

Figure 4–6
Metacarpals. This x-ray of a hand shows metacarpals, carpals (wrist bones), and phalanges (finger bones).

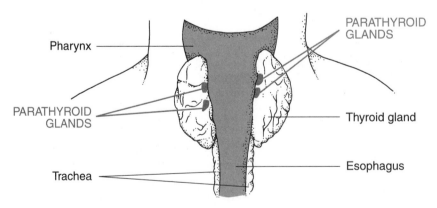

Figure 4–7
Parathyroid glands. These are four endocrine glands on the posterior (back side) of the thyroid gland.

paralysis _____
This term came from the Greek *paralyikos*, meaning "one whose side was loose or weak," as after a stroke. Now it means a loss of movement in any part of the body caused by a break in the connection between nerve and muscle.

paraplegia _____
-PLEGIA means paralysis and this term originally meant paralysis of any limb or side of the body. Since the 19th century, it indicates paralysis of the lower half of the body.

peri-	surrounding	periosteum _____
		perianal _____
poly-	many, much	polyuria _____
post-	after, behind	post partum _____
		post mortem _____
pre-	before	precancerous _____
		prenatal _____
pro-	before, forward	prolapse _____ -LAPSE means "to slide." Figure 4–8 shows a prolapsed uterus.
pros-	before, forward	prosthesis _____ An artificial limb is a prosthesis. Figure 4–9 illustrates several types of prostheses. Figure 4–10 shows total hip replacement and total knee joint replacements.
quadri-	four	quadriplegia _____ Paralysis of all four limbs.

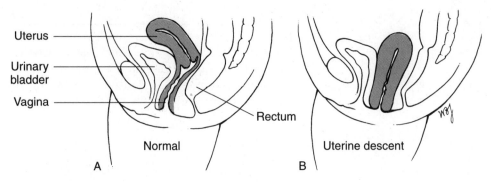

Uterus

Urinary
bladder

Vagina

Rectum

Normal

Uterine descent

A

B

Figure 4–8
Prolapsed uterus is shown in (B). Normally the uterus is tilted forward above the bladder (A).

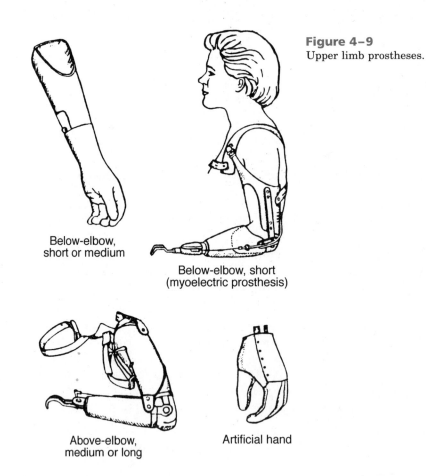

Below-elbow,
short or medium

Below-elbow, short
(myoelectric prosthesis)

Figure 4–9
Upper limb prostheses.

Above-elbow,
medium or long

Artificial hand

Figure 4–10

(A) Total hip joint replacement. A cementless prosthesis allows porous ingrowth of bone. (B) Total knee joint replacement using a tibial metal retainer and a femoral component. The femoral component is chosen individually for each person according to the amount of healthy bone present. (From Polaski AL and Tatro SE: Luckmann's Core Principles and Practice of Medical Surgical Nursing. Philadelphia, WB Saunders Co, 1996, with permission.)

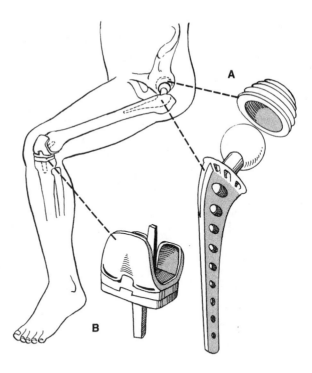

re-	back, behind	relapse _____ Symptoms of disease return. *Exacerbation* is an increase in the severity of a disease or any of its symptoms.
		remission _____ Symptoms of disease lessen.
		resection _____
retro-	back, behind	retroperitoneal _____ The kidneys and adrenal glands are retroperitoneal organs.
sub-	beneath, less than	subcostal _____
		subcutaneous _____

subtotal _____
A subtotal gastrectomy is a partial resection of the stomach.

subscapular _____
The scapula is the shoulder bone. Figure 4–11 shows its location.

syn-   with, together   syndrome _____
-DROME means "to run" or "occur." Syndromes are groups of symptoms or signs of illness that occur together. Table 4–3 gives examples of syndromes.

tachy-   fast   tachycardia _____

tachypnea _____

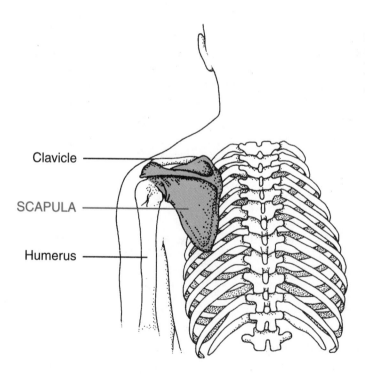

Figure 4–11
Scapula (shoulder bone), posterior view. The clavicle is the collar bone and the humerus is the upper arm bone.

Clavicle

SCAPULA

Humerus

TABLE 4–3.	SYNDROMES

Acquired immune deficiency syndrome (AIDS)
   Symptoms are severe infections, malignancy (Kaposi sarcoma and lymphoma), fever, malaise (discomfort), and gastrointestinal disturbances. It is caused by a virus that damages lymphocytes (white blood cells).

Barlow syndrome (mitral valve prolapse)
   Symptoms are abnormal sounds (murmurs) heard from the chest when listening with a stethoscope. These murmurs indicate that the mitral valve is not closing properly. Chest pain, dyspnea (difficult breathing), and fatigue are other symptoms.

Carpal tunnel syndrome
   Symptoms are pain, tingling, burning, and numbness of the hand. A nerve leading to the hand is compressed by connective tissue fibers in the wrist.

Down syndrome
   Symptoms include mental retardation, flat face with a short nose, slanted eyes, broad hands and feet, stubby fingers, and protruding lower lip. The syndrome occurs when an extra chromosome is present in each cell of the body.

Toxic shock syndrome
   Symptoms are high fever, vomiting, diarrhea, rash, hypotension (low blood pressure), and shock. It is caused by a bacterial infection in the vagina of menstruating women using superabsorbent tampons.

trans-	across, through	transabdominal _____
		transurethral _____
tri-	three	tricuspid valve _____
		CUSPID means "pointed end," as of a spear. The tricuspid valve is on the right side of the heart. The mitral or bicuspid valve is on the left side of the heart. Figure 4–12 shows the location of both valves and indicates the pathway of blood through the heart.
ultra-	beyond	ultrasonography _____
		Figure 4–13 shows an ultrasonogram (sonogram) of a 30-week fetus.
uni-	one	unilateral _____

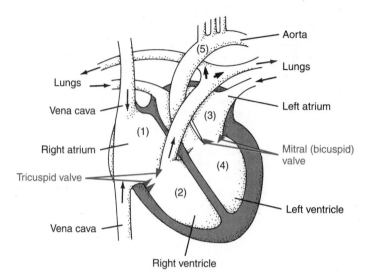

Figure 4–12

Tricuspid and mitral valves of the heart. Blood enters the *right atrium* of the heart (1) from the big veins (venae cavae) and passes through the *tricuspid valve* to the right ventricle (2). Blood then travels to the *lungs* where it loses carbon dioxide (a gaseous waste) and picks up oxygen. Blood returns to the heart into the *left atrium* (3) and passes through the mitral (bicuspid) valve to the *left ventricle* (4). It is then pumped from the left ventricle out the heart into the largest artery, the *aorta* (5), which carries the blood to all parts of the body.

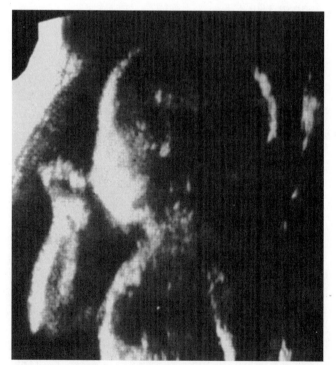

Figure 4–13

Ultrasonography. The 30-week fetus is sucking its thumb.

IV. Exercises

A.   Match the prefix in Column I with its meaning in Column II:

Column I	Column II

1. dia- ____	a. across, through
	b. no, not, without
2. neo- ____	c. bad, painful, difficult
	d. new
3. peri- ____	e. near, along the side of
	f. surrounding
4. an- ____	g. through, complete
	h. one
5. brady- ____	i. slow
	j. beyond
6. uni- ____	
7. trans- ____	
8. ultra- ____	
9. para- ____	
10. dys- ____	

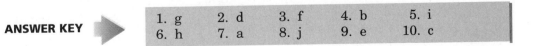

ANSWER KEY

1. g	2. d	3. f	4. b	5. i
6. h	7. a	8. j	9. e	10. c

B.   *Give meanings for the following prefixes:*

1.   meta- _____

2.   ana- _____

3.   a-, an- _____

4.   bi- _____

5.   inter- _____

6.   para- _____

7.   in- _____

8.   mal- _____

9.   anti- _____

10.   con- _____

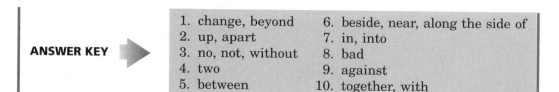

ANSWER KEY

1. change, beyond   6. beside, near, along the side of
2. up, apart   7. in, into
3. no, not, without   8. bad
4. two   9. against
5. between   10. together, with

C. *Select from the prefixes given in Column II to match meanings in Column I. Write the prefix in the space provided next to its meaning.*

Column I	Column II

1. bad, painful, difficult _____

2. out, outside, _____

3. away from _____

4. fast _____

5. before, forword _____

6. back, behind _____

7. less than, below _____

8. three _____

9. together, with _____

10. within _____

hyper-
meta-
pro-, pros-
intra-
syn-
ab-
re-, retro-
hypo-
uni-
dia-
tachy-
ec-
dys-
ad-
inter-
tri-

ANSWER KEY

1. dys-
2. ec-
3. ab-
4. tachy-
5. pro-, pros-

6. re-, retro-
7. hypo-
8. tri-
9. syn-
10. intra-

D. *Give meanings for the following prefixes:*

1. ante- _____

2. ad- _____

3. brady- _____

4. endo- _____

5. epi- _____

6. post- _____

7. pre- _____

8. sub- _____

9. extra- _____

10. dia- _____

11. hemi- _____

12. quadri- _____

ANSWER KEY ➤

1. before, forward	7. before
2. toward	8. beneath, less than
3. slow	9. out, outside of
4. within, in, inner	10. through, complete
5. above, upon	11. half
6. after, behind	12. four

E. Circle the meaning that is correct in each of the following:

1. Dys- and mal- both mean (outside, good, bad).
2. Hypo- and sub- both mean (below, above, outside).
3. Epi- and hyper- both mean (inside, beneath, above).
4. Con- and syn- both mean (apart, near, with).
5. Ultra- and meta- both mean (new, beyond, without).
6. Ante-, pre-, and pro- all mean (before, surrounding, between).
7. Ec- and extra- both mean (within, many, outside).

8. Endo-, intra-, and in- all mean (painful, within, through).

9. Post-, re-, and retro- all mean (behind, slow, together).

10. Uni- means (one, two, three).

11. Tri- means (one, two, three).

12. Bi- means (three, one, two).

ANSWER KEY ➡

1. bad	5. beyond	9. behind
2. below	6. before	10. one
3. above	7. outside	11. three
4. with	8. within	12. two

F. *Select from the following terms to complete the sentences below. The words in italics should be clues in your choice of the correct terms.*

analysis   prenatal   atrophy   unilateral
dysmenorrhea   bradycardia   adrenal glands   extracranial
antibody   dyspnea   parathyroid glands   epidural hematoma
bilateral   metacarpal   hypertrophy   antigen

1. Two glands located *near* (toward) the kidneys are the _____ .

2. People suffering from asthma often have *difficult* breathing, known as _____ .

3. A problem that only affects *one* side of the body is a(an) _____ defect.

4. Some people have a *slow* heart rhythm called _____ .

5. A condition of *painful* menstrual discharge is called _____ .

6. The bones that are *beyond* the wrist are the hand bones, or _____ bones.

7. A protein substance that is made by white blood cells *against* foreign

   microorganisms is called a(an) _____ .

8. An injury to the *outside* of the skull would be known as a(an) _____ lesion.

9. Four glands located in the neck region *near* (posterior to) another

endocrine gland are _____ .

10. Taking a substance *apart* to understand what it contains is called

a(an) _____ .

11. A collection of blood located *above* the outermost layer of membranes

surrounding the brain is called a(an) _____ .

12. A problem that occurs *before* the birth of an infant is called _____ .

13. *Excessive* development (individual cells increase in size) of an organ is known

as _____ .

14. When a part of the body is not used, *no* development occurs, and it shrinks

in size, known as _____ .

15. A problem affecting *both* sides of the body is called a(an) _____ defect.

ANSWER KEY ➤

1. adrenal glands	9. parathyroid glands
2. dyspnea	10. analysis
3. unilateral	11. epidural hematoma
4. bradycardia	12. prenatal
5. dysmenorrhea	13. hypertrophy
6. metacarpal	14. atrophy
7. antibody	15. bilateral
8. extracranial	

G. *Underline the prefix in each term, and give the meaning of the entire term:*

1. dysuria _____

2. hypoglycemia _____

3. intravenous _____

4. syndrome _____

5. precancerous _____

6. apnea _____

7. anemia _____

8. endoscopy _____

9. prosthesis _____

10. antibiotic _____

11. hemiplegia _____

12. dysphagia _____

ANSWER KEY ➤

1. dysuria—painful urination
2. hypoglycemia—low levels of sugar in the blood
3. intravenous—pertaining to within a vein
4. syndrome—group of symptoms that occur together, characterizing an abnormal condition
5. precancerous—before cancer
6. apnea—not breathing
7. anemia—literally, no blood; actually a decrease in red blood cells or in the hemoglobin within the cells
8. endoscopy—process of viewing within the body (an endoscope is used)
9. prosthesis—to put or place before (an artificial body part)
10. antibiotic—pertaining to a substance that is against bacterial or germ life
11. hemiplegia—paralysis of one half of the body
12. dysphagia—difficult swallowing

H. *Define the following terms that describe an organ, tissue, or space in the body:*

1. subscapular _____

2. intrauterine _____

3. periosteum _____

4. intervertebral _____

5. subcostal _____

6. transabdominal _____

7. perianal _____

8. extracranial _____

9. subcutaneous _____

10. retroperitoneal _____

ANSWER KEY ➤

1. under the shoulder
2. within the uterus
3. surrounding the bone (this is a membrane surrounding the bone)
4. between two vertebrae (a disk is an intervertebral structure)
5. under a rib
6. across the abdomen
7. surrounding the anus
8. outside the skull
9. under the skin
10. behind the peritoneum

I. *Use the following terms to fill in the blanks in the sentences below:*

congenital	ectopic	subtotal	metastasis
transurethral	prosthesis	malignant	hyperthyroidism
tachycardia	ultrasonography	tricuspid	endocrine
dialysis	diarrhea	dysplasia	antigen

1. Enlargement of an endocrine gland in the neck can lead to _____ .

2. An artificial limb is a(an) _____ .

3. If the colon does not reabsorb the proper amount of water back into the

   bloodstream, _____ occurs.

4. An abnormally rapid heart beat is a _____ .

5. Infection or abnormal ("bad") growth of cells on the uterine cervix can cause

   a condition known as cervical _____ .

6. A test that shows the structure of organs in the abdomen by using sound

   waves is _____ .

7. The spread of a cancerous tumor to a secondary place in the body is

   a(an) _____ .

8. The process of filtering the waste materials from the blood using a machine

   that does the work of the kidneys is called _____ .

9. The _____ valve is composed of three parts and is located on
   the right side of the heart between the upper and lower chambers.

10. A procedure to remove the prostate gland by cutting across (through) the

     urethra is a _____ resection of the prostate.

11. Cancerous growths are _____ neoplasms.

12. An abnormal condition that occurs at birth is a(an) _____
     anomaly.

13. A gland that secretes hormones into the bloodstream is a(an) _____
     gland.

14. A foreign organism, such as a virus or bacterium, that enters the body and

     stimulates white blood cells to make antibodies, is a(an) _____.

15. An embryo that grows outside the uterus (extrauterine) is a(an) _____
     pregnancy.

16. The doctors did not remove the whole organ; they did a partial or _____
     resection.

ANSWER KEY ➤

1. hyperthyroidism	9. tricuspid
2. prosthesis	10. transurethral
3. diarrhea	11. malignant
4. tachycardia	12. congenital
5. dysplasia	13. endocrine
6. ultrasonography	14. antigen
7. metastasis	15. ectopic
8. dialysis	16. subtotal

J.   Use the following terms to complete the sentences below:

transurethral	relapse	incision	analysis
prolapse	neoplastic	post partum	paralysis
neonatal	tachycardia	post mortem	anemia
remission	aphasia	ante partum	resection

1. Complete removal of Ms. Smith's stomach was necessary because of the

   presence of an adenocarcinoma. Dr. Nife performed the gastric _____.

2. After she had nine children, Ms. White's uterine walls became weak, causing

   her uterus to fall and _____ through her vagina.

3. The autopsy or _____ examination of a dead body is an
   important step in determining the cause of death.

4. After Mr. Puffer's heart attack, doctors were concerned because he continued
   to have a persistent, rapid, abnormal heart rhythm. They prescribed drugs

   called antiarrhythmics to treat his _____.

5. The special ward in the hospital devoted to newborn babies is known as the

   _____ unit.

6. Ms. Rose was pleased that she hadn't had symptoms of her malignant

   disease for the past six years. Her illness was in _____.

7. The operation to remove part of Mr. Jones' enlarged (hypertrophied) prostate
   gland involved placing a catheter through his urethra and removing pieces of

   the prostate through the tube. The surgery is called a _____
   resection of the prostate gland (TURP). The prostate gland is located at the
   base of the bladder in males. See Figure 4–14.

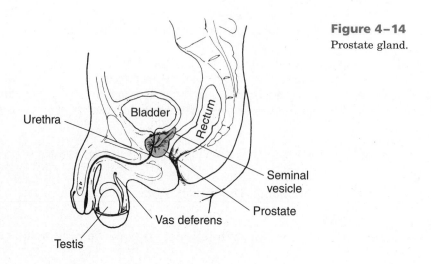

Figure 4–14
Prostate gland.

8. Mr. M. Pathy was in a sad mood for several weeks after his wife had their

   first baby. He was experiencing a(an) _____ depression.

9. Ms. Smith's recent stroke left her with loss of muscle movement on the right

   side of her body, also called right-sided _____.

10. Excessive bleeding or lack of iron in diet can lead to a decrease of hemoglobin

    in red blood cells, a condition known as iron-deficiency _____.

11. A CVA on the left side of the brain can cause a deficit or loss of speech,

    known as _____.

ANSWER KEY ➡

1. resection
2. prolapse
3. post mortem
4. tachycardia
5. neonatal
6. remission
7. transurethral
8. post partum
9. paralysis
10. anemia
11. aphasia

K. *Circle the term that best completes the meaning of the sentences in the following medical vignettes:*

1. As part of her (**intravenous, post partum, antenatal**) care, Bea underwent (**ultrasonography, endoscopy, urinalysis**) to determine the fetal age and to make sure that there were no anatomical anomalies.

2. Ellen's pregnancy test was positive but she had excruciating pelvic pain. After an examination and ultrasound, the doctors diagnosed a(an) (**epidural, ectopic, subscapular**) pregnancy. She then had emergency surgery to remove the early pregnancy from the fallopian tube.

3. After noticing a suspicious-looking mole on her upper arm, Carole was diagnosed with (**malignant, benign, subtotal**) melanoma. This type of skin cancer is a(an) (**intrauterine, extrahepatic, neoplastic**) process and has a high likelihood of (**paralysis, dysplasia, metastasis**) to other areas of the body.

4. Carole's daughter, Annabelle, found a mole on her back and quickly had it checked out by her physician. Fortunately, after a biopsy, the pathology revealed a (**transabdominal, precancerous, perianal**) nevus (mole) that was considered (**chronic, unilateral, benign**). In the future, she would need close follow-up for other suspicious lesions.

5. Milton's blood pressure was 160/110. Normal blood pressure is 120/80. Because of his (**bradycardia, hypertension, dyspnea**), Milton's physician prescribed medication to reduce his risk of stroke.

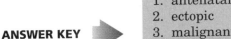

ANSWER KEY

1. antenatal, ultrasonography
2. ectopic
3. malignant, neoplastic, metastasis
4. precancerous, benign
5. hypertension

V. Review

Write the meanings for the following word parts, and please don't forget to check your answers.

PREFIXES

Prefix	Meaning	Prefix	Meaning
1. a-, an-	_____	20. inter-	_____
2. ab-	_____	21. intra-	_____
3. ad-	_____	22. mal-	_____
4. ana-	_____	23. meta-	_____
5. ante-	_____	24. neo-	_____
6. anti-	_____	25. para-	_____
7. bi-	_____	26. peri-	_____
8. brady-	_____	27. post-	_____
9. con-	_____	28. pre-	_____
10. dia-	_____	29. pro-, pros-	_____
11. dys-	_____	30. quadri-	_____
12. ec-	_____	31. re-, retro-	_____
13. endo-	_____	32. sub-	_____
14. epi-	_____	33. syn-	_____
15. ex-, extra-	_____	34. tachy-	_____
16. hemi-	_____	35. trans-	_____
17. hyper-	_____	36. tri-	_____
18. hypo-	_____	37. ultra-	_____
19. in-	_____	38. uni-	_____

COMBINING FORMS

Combining Form	Meaning	Combining Form	Meaning
1. abdomin/o	_____	16. norm/o	_____
2. an/o	_____	17. oste/o	_____
3. bi/o	_____	18. peritone/o	_____
4. cardi/o	_____	19. plas/o	_____
5. carp/o	_____	20. ren/o	_____
6. cis/o	_____	21. scapul/o	_____
7. cost/o	_____	22. son/o	_____
8. crani/o	_____	23. thyroid/o	_____
9. cutane/o	_____	24. top/o	_____
10. dur/o	_____	25. troph/o	_____
11. gen/o	_____	26. urethr/o	_____
12. glyc/o	_____	27. uter/o	_____
13. hemat/o	_____	28. ven/o	_____
14. later/o	_____	29. vertebr/o	_____
15. nat/i	_____		

SUFFIXES

Suffix	Meaning	Suffix	Meaning
1. -al	_____	15. -ous	_____
2. -ation	_____	16. -partum	_____
3. -cision	_____	17. -plasm	_____
4. -crine	_____	18. -pnea	_____
5. -emia	_____	19. -rrhea	_____
6. -gen	_____	20. -scopy	_____
7. -graphy	_____	21. -section	_____
8. -ia	_____	22. -stasis	_____
9. -ic	_____	23. -tension	_____
10. -ine	_____	24. -thesis	_____
11. -ism	_____	25. -tic	_____
12. -lysis	_____	26. -um	_____
13. -mortem	_____	27. -uria	_____
14. -oma	_____	28. -y	_____

PREFIXES

1. no, not, without
2. away from
3. toward
4. up, apart
5. before, forward
6. against
7. two
8. slow
9. with, together
10. through, complete
11. bad, painful, difficult
12. out, outside
13. within, in, inner
14. above, upon
15. out, outside
16. half
17. excessive, above
18. below, under
19. in, into
20. between
21. within
22. bad
23. change, beyond
24. new
25. beside, near, along the side of
26. surrounding
27. after, behind
28. before
29. before, forward
30. four
31. back, behind
32. beneath, less than
33. with, together
34. fast
35. across, through
36. three
37. beyond
38. one

COMBINING FORMS

1. abdomen
2. anus
3. life
4. heart
5. wrist bones
6. to cut
7. ribs
8. skull
9. skin
10. dura mater
11. to produce
12. sugar
13. blood
14. side
15. birth
16. rule, order
17. bone
18. peritoneum
19. formation, growth
20. kidney
21. shoulder blade (bone)
22. sound
23. thyroid gland
24. to put, place
25. development, nourishment
26. urethra
27. uterus
28. vein
29. vertebra (backbone)

SUFFIXES

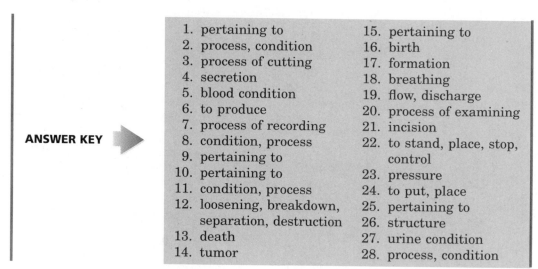

ANSWER KEY

1. pertaining to
2. process, condition
3. process of cutting
4. secretion
5. blood condition
6. to produce
7. process of recording
8. condition, process
9. pertaining to
10. pertaining to
11. condition, process
12. loosening, breakdown, separation, destruction
13. death
14. tumor
15. pertaining to
16. birth
17. formation
18. breathing
19. flow, discharge
20. process of examining
21. incision
22. to stand, place, stop, control
23. pressure
24. to put, place
25. pertaining to
26. structure
27. urine condition
28. process, condition

VI. Pronunciation of Terms

The terms that you have learned in this chapter are presented here with their pronunciations. The capitalized letters in boldface are the accented syllable. Pronounce each word out loud, then write the meaning in the space provided.

Term	Pronunciation	Meaning
abnormal	ab-**NOR**-mal	_____
adrenal glands	ad-**RE**-nal glanz	_____
analysis	ah-**NAL**-ih-sis	_____
anemia	ah-**NE**-me-ah	_____
ante mortem	**AN**-te **MOR**-tem	_____
ante partum	**AN**-te **PAR**-tum	_____

antenatal	**AN**-te **NA**-tal _____
antibiotic	an-tih-bi-**OT**-ik _____
antibodies	an-tih-**BOD**-eez _____
antigen	**AN**-tih-jen _____
aphasia	a-**FA**-ze-ah _____
apnea	**AP**-ne-ah _____
atrophy	**AT**-ro-fe _____
benign	Be-**NIN** _____
bilateral	bi-**LAT**-er-al _____
bradycardia	bra-de-**KAR**-de-ah _____
congenital anomaly	kon-**JEN**-ih-tal ah-**NOM**-ah-le _____
dialysis	di-**AL**-ih-sis _____
diarrhea	di-ah-**RE**-ah _____
dysphagia	dis-**FA**-jah _____
dysplasia	dis-**PLA**-se-ah _____
dyspnea	**DISP**-ne-ah _____
dysuria	dis-**U**-re-ah _____
ectopic pregnancy	ek-**TOP**-ik **PREG**-nan-se _____

endocrine glands	**EN**-do-krin glanz _____
endoscopy	en-**DOS**-ko-pe _____
epidural hematoma	ep-ih-**DUR**-al he-mah-**TO**-mah _____
excision	ek-**SIZH**-un _____
extrahepatic	eks-tra-heh-**PAT**-ik _____
hemigastrectomy	heh-me-gas-**TREK**-to-me _____
hemiplegia	heh-me-**PLE**-jah _____
hypeglycemia	hi-per-gli-**SE**-me-ah _____
hypertension	hi-per-**TEN**-shun _____
hyperthyroidism	hi-per-**THI**-royd-izm _____
hypertrophy	hi-**PER**-tro-fe _____
hypoglycemia	hi-po-gli-**SE**-me-ah _____
incision	in-**SIZH**-un _____
intervertebral	in-ter-**VER**-teh-bral _____
intrauterine	in-tra-**U**-ter-in _____
intravenous	in-trah-**VE**-nus _____
malignant	mah-**LIG**-nant _____
metacarpal	met-ah-**KAR**-pal _____

metastasis	meh-**TAS**-tah-sis
neonatal	ne-o-**NA**-tal
neoplastic	ne-o-**PLAS**-tik
paralysis	pah-**RAL**-ih-sis
paraplegia	par-ah-**PLE**-jah
parathyroid glands	par-ah-**THI**-royd glanz
perianal	per-e-**A**-nal
periosteum	per-e-**OS**-te-um
polyuria	pol-e-**UR**-e-ah
post mortem	post **MOR**-tem
part partum	post **PAR**-tum
precancerous	pre-**KAN**-ser-us
prolapse	pro-**LAPS**
prosthesis	pros-**THE**-sis
quadriplegia	quah-drah-**PLE**-jah
relapse	re-**LAPS**
remission	re-**MISH**-un
resection	re-**SEK**-shun

retroperitoneal	reh-tro-peri-ih-to-**NE**-al _____
subcostal	sub-**KOS**-tal _____
subcutaneous	sub-ku-**TA**-ne-us _____
subdural hematoma	sub-**DUR**-al he-mah-**TO**-mah _____
subscapular	sub-**SKAP**-u-lar _____
subtotal	sub-**TO**-tal _____
syndrome	**SIN**-drom _____
tachycardia	tak-eh-**KAR**-de-ah _____
tachypnea	tak-ip-**NE**-ah _____
transabdominal	trans-ab-**DOM**-ih-nal _____
transurethral	trans-u-**RE**-thral _____
tricuspid valve	tri-**KUS**-id valv _____
ultrasonography	ul-trah-son-**OG**-rah-fe _____
unilateral	u-nih-**LAT**-er-al _____
urinalysis	u-rih-**NAL**-ih-sis _____

VII. Practical Applications

A. *Match the abnormal condition in Column I with the organ lesion or body part in Column II that may be the cause of the condition:*

Column I		Column II
1. aphasia	_____	A. urinary bladder
		B. colon
2. dysphagia	_____	C. uterine cervix
		D. left-sided brain lesion
3. diarrhea	_____	E. pancreas
		F. lungs
4. quadriplegia	_____	G. heart
		H. cervical spinal cord lesion
5. hyperglycemia	_____	I. esophagus
		J. lumbar spinal cord lesion
6. dysuria	_____	
7. paraplegia	_____	
8. bradycardia	_____	
9. dyspnea	_____	
10. dysplasia	_____	

ANSWER KEY
1. D   2. I   3. B   4. H   5. E
6. A   7. J   8. G   9. F   10. C

(Continued)

B. Pathology: Disease description—HYPERTHYROIDISM
    From the following terms complete the sentences in the paragraph below:

bradycardia	hypersecretion	hyposecretion	hypoplastic
dyspnea	antibodies	antibiotics	goiter
tachycardia	hyperplastic	exophthalmia	neoplastic

Hyperthyroidism, also known as thyrotoxicosis or Graves disease, is marked by an excess of thyroid hormones. There is much evidence to support a hereditary factor in the development of this condition and some consider it an

autoimmune disorder caused by _____ that bind to the surface of

thyroid gland cells and stimulate _____ of hormones (T_3 and T_4—triiodothyronine and thyroxine). The enlarged gland, histologically, is composed

of _____ follicles lined with hyperactive cells.

Symptoms of hyperthyroidism include restlessness, insomnia, weight loss,

sweating, and rapid heartbeat or _____. Abnormal protrusion of

the eyes, known as _____, is another symptom. The patient also

presents with an enlarged thyroid gland, called a _____.

ANSWER KEY ➤ antibodies
hypersecretion
hyperplastic
tachycardia
exophthalmia
goiter

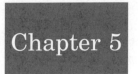

Medical Specialists and Case Reports

C H A P T E R   O B J E C T I V E S

- To describe the training process of physicians
- To identify medical specialists and describe their specialties
- To identify combining forms used in terms that describe specialists
- To decipher medical terminology as written in case reports

153

I. Introduction

This chapter reviews many of the terms you have learned in previous chapters while adding others related to medical specialists. In Section II, the training of physicians is described and specialists are listed with their specialties. Section III uses combining forms, which are found in the terms describing specialists, with familiar suffixes to test your knowledge of terms. In Section IV, short case reports are presented to illustrate the use of the medical language in context. As you read these reports, you will be impressed with your ability to understand medical terminology!

II. Medical Specialists

Doctors complete four years of medical school and, after passing National Medical Board Examinations, receive an M.D. (Medical Doctor) degree. They may then begin post-graduate training, the length of which is at least three years, and in some cases longer. This postgraduate training is known as *residency training*. Examples of residency programs are:

Anesthesiology	Administration of agents capable of bringing about a loss of sensation
Dermatology	Diagnosis and treatment of skin disorders
Emergency medicine	Care of patients that requires sudden and immediate action
Family practice	Primary care of all members of the family on a continuing basis
Internal medicine	Diagnosis of disorders and treatment with drugs
Ophthalmology	Diagnosis and treatment of eye disorders
Pathology	Diagnosis of the cause and nature of disease
Pediatrics	Diagnosis and treatment of children's disorders
Psychiatry	Diagnosis and treatment of disorders of the mind
Radiology	Diagnosis using x-rays and other procedures (ultrasound and magnetic resonance imaging)
Surgery	Treatment by manual (surg- means hand) or operative methods

Examinations are administered after completion of each residency program to certify competency in that specialty area.

A physician may then choose to specialize further by doing *fellowship* training. Fellowships (two to five years) train doctors in *clinical* (patient care) and *research* (laboratory) skills. For example, an *internist* (specialist in internal medicine) may choose fellowship training in internal medicine specialties such as neurology, nephrology, endocrinology, and oncology. A surgeon interested in further specialization may do fellowship training in thoracic surgery, neurosurgery, or plastic surgery. Upon completion of training and examinations, the doctor is then a recognized specialist in that specialty area.

Medical specialists and an explanation of their specialties are listed below:

Medical Specialist	Specialty
allergist	Treatment of hypersensitivity reactions
anesthesiologist	Administration of agents for loss of sensation
cardiologist	Treatment of heart disease
cardiovascular surgeon	Surgery on the heart and blood vessels
colorectal surgeon	Surgery on the colon and rectum
dermatologist	Treatment of skin disorders
emergency physician	Immediate evaluation and treatment for people with acute injury and illness in a hospital setting
endocrinologist	Treatment of endocrine gland disorders
family physician	Primary care and treatment of families on a continuing basis
gastroenterologist	Treatment of stomach and intestinal disorders
geriatrician	Treatment of diseases of old age
gynecologist	Surgery and treatment of the female reproductive system
hematologist	Treatment of blood disorders
infectious disease specialist	Treatment of diseases caused by microorganisms
internist	Provide comprehensive care to adults in an office or hospital
nephrologist	Treatment of kidney diseases
neurologist	Treatment of nerve disorders
neurosurgeon	Surgery on the brain, spinal cord, and nerves
obstetrician	Treatment of pregnant women; delivery of babies
oncologist	Diagnosis and medical treatment of malignant and benign tumors
ophthalmologist	Surgical and medical treatment of eye disorders
orthopedist	Surgical treatment of bones, muscles, and joints
otolaryngologist	Treatment of the ear, nose, and throat
pathologist	Diagnosis of disease by analysis of cells
pediatrician	Treatment of diseases of children
physical medicine and rehabilitation specialist	Treatment to restore function after illness
psychiatrist	Treatment of mental disorders
pulmonary specialist	Treatment of lung diseases

radiologist	Examination of x-rays to determine a diagnosis; includes interpretation of ultrasound images and MRI and nuclear medicine as well
radiation oncologist	Treatment of disease with high-energy radiation
rheumatologist	Treatment of joint and muscle disorders
thoracic surgeon	Surgery on chest organs
urologist	Surgery on the urinary tract

III. Combining Forms and Vocabulary

The combining forms listed below are familiar because they are found in the terms describing medical specialists. A medical term is included to illustrate the use of the combining form. Write the meaning of the medical term in the space provided. You can always check your answers with the glossary at the end of the book.

Combining Form	Meaning	Medical Term	Meaning
cardi/o	heart	cardiomegaly	_____
col/o	colon	colostomy	_____
dermat/o	skin	dermatitis	_____
endocrin/o	endocrine glands	endocrinology	_____
enter/o	intestines	enteritis	_____
esthesi/o	sensation	anesthesiology	_____
gastr/o	stomach	gastroscopy	_____
ger/o	old age	geriatrics	_____
gynec/o	woman, female	gynecology	_____

hemat/o	blood	hematoma _____

iatr/o   treatment   iatrogenic _____
IATR/O means treatment by a physician or with medicines. An iatrogenic illness is *produced* (-genic) unexpectedly by a treatment.

laryng/o   voice box   laryngeal _____

nephr/o   kidney   nephrostomy _____

neur/o   nerve   neuralgia _____

nos/o   disease   nosocomial _____
A nosocomial infection is aquired during hospitalization (comi/o means to care for).

obstetr/o   midwife   obstetric _____

onc/o   tumor   oncogenic _____
Oncogenic viruses give rise to tumors.

ophthalm/o   eye   ophthalmologist _____

opt/o   eye   optometrist _____
An optometrist examines (METR means "measure") eyes and prescribes glasses but cannot treat eye diseases.

optician _____
Opticians grind lenses and fit glasses but do not examine eyes, prescribe glasses, or treat eye diseases.

orth/o   straight   orthopedist _____
PED/O comes from the Greek, *paidos*, meaning "child." Orthopedists in the past were concerned with straightening bone deformities in children.

ot/o	ear	otitis _____
path/o	disease	pathology _____
ped/o	child	pediatrics _____
psych/o	mind	psychosis _____
pulmon/o	lung	pulmonary _____
radi/o	x-rays	radiotherapy _____ Also called radiation therapy.
rect/o	rectum	rectocele _____ -CELE means "a hernia or protrusion." The walls of the rectum weaken and bulge forward toward the vagina. See Figure 5–1.
rheumat/o	flow, fluid	rheumatology _____ Joints can fill with fluid when diseased, hence RHEUMAT/O indicates a problem with a swollen joint. Rheumatoid arthritis is a chronic inflammatory disease of joints and connective tissues which leads to deformation of joints. See Figure 5–2.

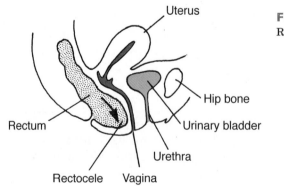

Figure 5–1
Rectocele.

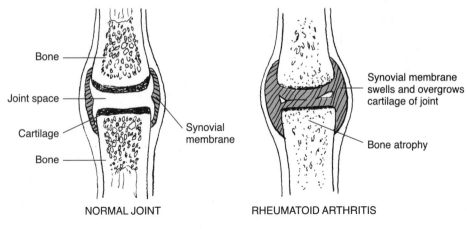

Figure 5–2
Normal joint and rheumatoid arthritis.

rhin/o	nose	rhinorrhea _____
thorac/o	chest	thoracotomy _____
ur/o	urinary tract	urology _____
vascul/o	blood vessels	vasculitis _____

IV. Case Reports

Here are short reports related to medical specialties. Many terms are familiar, others are explained in the glossary. Write the meaning of the boldface term in the space provided.

CASE 1 | CARDIOLOGY

Mr. Rose was admitted to the Cardiac Care Unit (CCU) following a severe **myocardial infarction**. He had suffered from **angina** (due to **ischemia**), and **hypertension** for some time previously. He is being treated with

antiarrhythmic drugs, **diuretics**, and **anticoagulants**. If his recovery proceeds as expected, he will be discharged in three weeks.

angina _____

antiarrhythmic _____

anticoagulant _____

diuretic _____

hypertension _____

ischemia _____

myocardial infarction _____

CASE 2 | **GYNECOLOGY**

Ms. Sessions has been complaining of **dysmenorrhea** and **menorrhagia** for several months. She is also **anemic**. Because of the presence of large **fibroids**, as seen on a pelvic **ultrasound** exam (**sonogram**), **hysterectomy** is recommended.

anemic _____

dysmenorrhea _____

fibroids _____

hysterectomy _____

menorrhagia _____

sonogram _____

ultrasound _____

CASE 3 | **ONCOLOGY**

The patient is a 26-year-old female with a previous diagnosis of **mediastinal** and **intra-abdominal Hodgkin disease**. She is admitted to the hospital for **lymphangiography** and **percutaneous** liver **biopsy** after discovery of possible recurrence of tumor.

Following the assessment of her **platelet** count, a percutaneous liver biopsy was performed and showed normal **hepatic** tissue. The **lymphangiogram** was normal as well. The patient was later scheduled for **peritoneoscopy**.

biopsy _____

hepatic _____

Hodgkin disease _____

intra-abdominal _____

lymphangiogram _____

lymphangiography _____

mediastinal _____

percutaneous _____

peritoneoscopy _____

platelet _____

CASE 4 | **UROLOGY**

Polly Smith has a history of lower back pain associated with **hematuria** and **dysuria**. She has an appointment at the hospital for investigation of her symptoms. Tests include an **intravenous pyelogram** (IVP) and **cystoscopy**.

    The findings of these tests confirm the diagnosis of **renal calculus**. **Lithotripsy** is recommended and **prognosis** is favorable.

calculus _____

cystoscopy _____

dysuria _____

hematuria _____

intravenous pyelogram (IVP) _____

lithotripsy _____

prognosis _____

renal _____

CASE 5 | **GASTROENTEROLOGY**

Mr. Pepper suffers from **dyspepsia** and sharp **abdominal** pain. A recent episode of **hematemesis** has left him very weak and **anemic**.

    Gastroscopy and **barium swallow** revealed the presence of a large **ulcer**. He will be admitted to the hospital and scheduled for a partial **gastrectomy**.

abdominal _____

anemic _____

barium swallow _____

dyspepsia _____

gastrectomy _____

gastroscopy _____

hematemesis _____

ulcer _____

CASE 6 | **RADIOLOGY**

Examination: **Thoracic cavity**. PA (**posterior-anterior**) and **lateral** chest. There is a patchy **infiltrate** in the right lower **lobe** seen best in the lateral view. The heart and **mediastinal** structures are normal. No evidence of **pleural effusion**.
   Impression: Right lower lobe **pneumonia**

anterior _____

infiltrate _____

lateral _____

lobe _____

mediastinal _____

pleural effusion _____

pneumonia _____

posterior _____

thoracic cavity _____

CASE 7 | **ORTHOPEDICS**

A 20-year-old male patient was admitted to the hospital following a motorcycle accident. In the accident he sustained **fractures** of the right **tibia**, right **femur**, and **pelvis** and **intra-abdominal** injuries.

Two pins were placed through the lower and upper end of the tibia and a cast was applied. Two days later he was taken to surgery and internal **fixation** of the right femur was performed.

femur _____

fixation _____

fracture _____

intra-abdominal _____

pelvis _____

tibia _____

CASE 8 | **NEPHROLOGY**

A 52-year-old man with **chronic renal failure** secondary to long-standing **hypertension** has been maintained on **hemodialysis** for the past 18 months. For the past three weeks during the dialysis sessions he has become moderately **hypotensive**, with symptoms of dizziness. Consequently, we have decided to withhold his **antihypertensive** medications prior to dialysis.

antihypertensive _____

chronic _____

hemodialysis _____

hypertension _____

hypotensive _____

renal failure _____

CASE 9 | **ENDOCRINOLOGY**

A 36-year-old woman known to have **insulin**-dependent **diabetes mellitus** (type I) was brought to the emergency room after being found collapsed in her home. She had experienced three days of extreme weakness, **polyuria**, and **polydipsia**. It was discovered that a few days prior to her admission she had discontinued her insulin in a suicide attempt.

diabetes mellitus _____

insulin _____

polydipsia _____

polyuria _____

CASE 10 | **NEUROLOGY**

Ms. Rose is admitted with severe, throbbing **unilateral frontal cephalgia** that has lasted for two days. Light makes her cringe and she complains of **nausea**. Before the onset of these symptoms, she saw zigzag lines for about 20 minutes. Diagnosis is **acute migraine** with **aura**. A **vasoconstrictor** is prescribed, and Ms. Rose's condition is improving. (Migraine headaches are thought to be caused by sudden **dilation** of blood vessels.)

acute _____

aura _____

cephalgia _____

dilation _____

frontal _____

migraine _____

nausea _____

unilateral _____

vasoconstrictor _____

V. Exercises

These exercises test your understanding of the terms in Sections II and III. Don't forget to check your responses with the answers directly following each exercise.

A.   Match the following residency programs with their descriptions that follow:

internal medicine   pediatrics   psychiatry
radiology   surgery   family practice
anesthesiology   emergency medicine   pathology
dermatology   ophthalmology

1.   Treatment by operation or manual (hand) methods: _____

2.   Diagnosis of adult disorders and treatment with drugs: _____

3.   Diagnosis and treatment of disorders of the mind: _____

4.   Primary care of all family members on a continuing basis: _____

5. Diagnosis and treatment of skin disorders: _____

6. Diagnosis and treatment of eye disorders: _____

7. Diagnosis of disease using x-rays: _____

8. Diagnosis and treatment of children's disorders: _____

9. Care of patients that requires immediate action: _____

10. Administration of agents that cause loss of sensation: _____

11. Diagnosis of disease by examining cells and tissues: _____

ANSWER KEY ➡

1. surgery	7. radiology
2. internal medicine	8. pediatrics
3. psychiatry	9. emergency medicine
4. family practice	10. anesthesiology
5. dermatology	11. pathology
6. ophthalmology	

B. Name the doctor who treats the following problems (first letters are given):

1. Kidney diseases   N _____

2. Tumors   O _____

3. Broken bones   O _____

4. Female diseases   G _____

5. Eye disorders   O _____

6. Heart disorders   C _____

7. Nerve disorders   N _____

8. Lung disorders   P _____

9. Mental disorders   P _____

10. Stomach and intestinal disorders   G _____

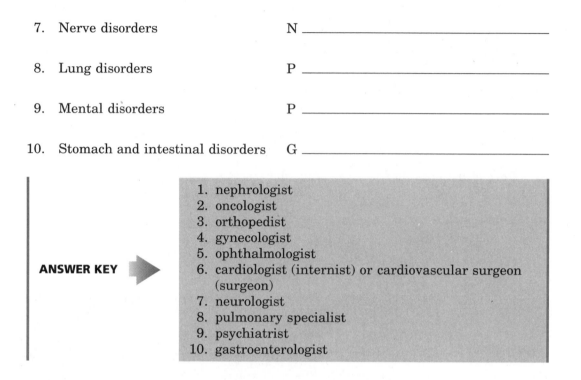

ANSWER KEY ➤

1. nephrologist
2. oncologist
3. orthopedist
4. gynecologist
5. ophthalmologist
6. cardiologist (internist) or cardiovascular surgeon (surgeon)
7. neurologist
8. pulmonary specialist
9. psychiatrist
10. gastroenterologist

C. *Match the following medical specialists in Column I with their specialties in Column II:*

Column I	Column II

Column I

1. urologist   _____

2. thoracic surgeon   _____

3. radiation oncologist _____

4. colorectal surgeon _____

5. endocrinologist   _____

6. obstetrician   _____

Column II

A. Operates on the large intestine
B. Treats blood disorders
C. Treats thyroid and pituitary gland disorders
D. Delivers babies
E. Treats children and their disorders
F. Operates on the urinary tract
G. Treats disorders of the skin
H. Treats tumors by using high-energy radiation
I. Operates on the chest
J. Examines x-rays to diagnose disease

7. radiologist   ——

8. pediatrician   ——

9. hematologist   ——

10. dermatologist   ——

D.   Complete the sentences that follow using the terms listed below:

clinical   orthopedist   optometrist   infectious disease specialist
pathologist   optician   research   geriatrician
ophthalmologist   oncologist   surgeon

1. A physician who diagnoses and treats diseases that are caused by

    microorganisms is a(an) ——————————————————————.

2. A doctor who does bone surgery is a(an) ——————————————.

3. A doctor who takes care of patients does —————————————— medicine.

4. A person who grinds lenses and fills prescriptions for eye glasses is a(an)

    ————————————————————————————————.

5. A doctor who reads biopsy samples and performs autopsies is a(an)

    ————————————————————————————————.

6. A doctor who treats cancerous tumors is a(an) ——————————.

7. A person who can examine eyes and prescribe eye glasses but cannot treat

   eye disorders is a(an) _____ .

8. A doctor who operates on patients is a(an) _____ .

9. A doctor who does experiments with test tubes and laboratory equipment is

   interested in _____ medicine.

10. A doctor who specializes in treatment of disorders of the eye is a(an)

    _____ .

11. A doctor who specializes in the treatment of older people is a(an)

    _____ .

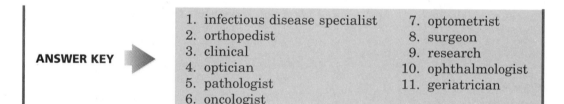

ANSWER KEY

1. infectious disease specialist
2. orthopedist
3. clinical
4. optician
5. pathologist
6. oncologist
7. optometrist
8. surgeon
9. research
10. ophthalmologist
11. geriatrician

E. *Which medical specialist would you consult for the following medical conditions? The first letter of the specialist is given.*

1. Arthritis   R _____

2. Otitis media   O _____

3. Anemia   H _____

4. Urinary bladder displacement   U _____

5. Chronic bronchitis   P _____

6. Cerebrovascular accident   N _____

7. Breast cancer   O _____

8. Hole in the wall of the heart   C _____

9. Dislocated shoulder bone   O _____

10. Thyroid gland enlargement   E _____

11. Kidney disease   N _____

12. Acne (skin disorder)   D _____

13. Hay fever (hypersensitivity reaction)   A _____

14. Viral and bacterial diseases   I _____

ANSWER KEY ➡

1. rheumatologist
2. otolaryngologist
3. hematologist
4. urologist
5. pulmonary specialist
6. neurologist
7. oncologist
8. cardiovascular surgeon
9. orthopedist
10. endocrinologist
11. nephrologist
12. dermatologist
13. allergist
14. infectious disease specialist

F.　*Give meanings for the following medical terms:*

1.　neuralgia _____

2.　pathology _____

3.　cardiomegaly _____

4.　nephrostomy _____

5.　thoracotomy _____

6.　laryngeal _____

7.　otitis _____

8.　colostomy _____

9.　pulmonary _____

10.　iatrogenic _____

11.　gastroscopy _____

12.　radiotherapy _____

13.　anesthesiology _____

14.　enteritis _____

15.　nosocomial _____

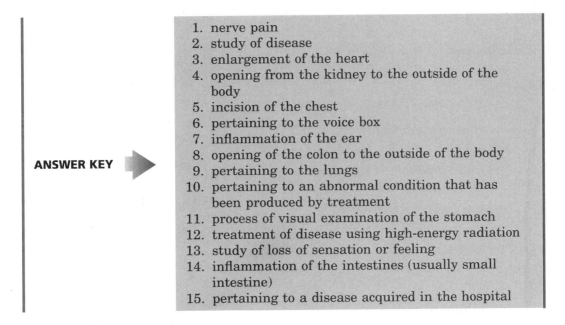

ANSWER KEY

1. nerve pain
2. study of disease
3. enlargement of the heart
4. opening from the kidney to the outside of the body
5. incision of the chest
6. pertaining to the voice box
7. inflammation of the ear
8. opening of the colon to the outside of the body
9. pertaining to the lungs
10. pertaining to an abnormal condition that has been produced by treatment
11. process of visual examination of the stomach
12. treatment of disease using high-energy radiation
13. study of loss of sensation or feeling
14. inflammation of the intestines (usually small intestine)
15. pertaining to a disease acquired in the hospital

G. *Use the following combining forms and suffixes to make the medical terms called for:*

Combining Forms		Suffixes	
laryng/o	nephr/o	-itis	-scopy
neur/o	ophthalm/o	-ectomy	-osis
onc/o	thorac/o	-tomy	-logy
col/o	ot/o	-algia	-therapy
psych/o	path/o	-genic	-stomy

1. Inflammation of the ear: _____

2. Removal of a nerve: _____

3. Incision of the chest: _____

4. Study of tumors: _____

5. Pertaining to producing disease: _____

6. Inflammation of the voice box: _____

7. Opening of the large intestine to the outside of the body: _____

8. Visual examination of the eye: _____

9. Abnormal condition of the mind: _____

10. Inflammation of the kidney: _____

11. Removal of the large intestine: _____

12. Pain in the ear: _____

13. Treatment of the mind: _____

14. Pertaining to producing tumors: _____

ANSWER KEY ➤	
1. otitis	8. ophthalmoscopy
2. neurectomy	9. psychosis
3. thoracotomy	10. nephritis
4. oncology	11. colectomy
5. pathogenic	12. otalgia
6. laryngitis	13. psychotherapy
7. colostomy	14. oncogenic

H. *Circle the term that best completes the meaning of the sentences in the following medical vignettes:*

1. Dr. Butler is a specialized physician who operates on hearts. He trained as a (**neurologic, cardiovascular, pulmonary**) surgeon. Often, his procedures require that Dr. Baker, a(an) (**gynecologic, ophthalmic, thoracic**) surgeon, assist him when the chest and lungs need surgical intervention.

2. Pauline noticed a rash over most of her body. First she saw Dr. Cole, her (**family practice doctor, oncologist, radiologist**) who performs her yearly physicals. Dr. Cole, who is not a(an) (**endocrinologist, orthopedist,**

dermatologist) by training, referred her to a skin specialist to make the proper diagnosis and treat the rash.

3. Dr. Liu is a(an) (**internist, obstetrician, pediatrician**) as well as a(an) (**nephrologist, urologist, gynecologist**), and can take care of her female patients before, during, and after their pregnancies.

4. After her sixth pregnancy, Sally developed an abnormal condition at the lower end of her colon. She went to a(an) (**gastroenterologist, hematologist, optometrist**), who made the diagnosis of protrusion of the rectum into the vagina. She then consulted colorectal and gynecologic surgeons to make an appropriate treatment plan for her condition, known as a (**vasculitis, rectocele, colostomy**).

5. In the cancer clinic, patients often must see a medical (**oncologist, orthopedist, rheumatologist**) who administers chemotherapy, and a(an) (**psychiatrist, radiation oncologist, radiologist**) who prescribes (**drugs, surgery, radiation therapy**) to treat tumors with high-energy protons and electrons.

6. While recovering from successful surgery in the hospital, Janet developed a cough and fever. Her surgeon ordered a chest x-ray and suspected a(an) (**oncogenic, nosocomial, iatrogenic**) pneumonia. A(an) (**anesthesiologist, neurologist, infectious disease specialist**) was called in to diagnose and treat the hospital-acquired disease condition.

ANSWER KEY ➡

1. cardiovascular, thoracic
2. family practice doctor, dermatologist
3. obstetrician, gynecologist
4. gastroenterologist, rectocele
5. oncologist, radiation oncologist, radiation therapy
6. nosocomial, infectious disease specialist

VI. Review

Test your understanding of the combining forms and suffixes in this chapter by completing the following review exercise:

COMBINING FORMS

Combining Form	Meaning	Combining Form	Meaning
1. cardi/o	_____	17. onc/o	_____
2. col/o	_____	18. ophthalm/o	_____
3. dermat/o	_____	19. opt/o	_____
4. endocrin/o	_____	20. orth/o	_____
5. enter/o	_____	21. ot/o	_____
6. esthesi/o	_____	22. path/o	_____
7. gastr/o	_____	23. ped/o	_____
8. ger/o	_____	24. psych/o	_____
9. gynec/o	_____	25. pulmon/o	_____
10. hemat/o	_____	26. radi/o	_____
11. iatr/o	_____	27. rect/o	_____
12. laryng/o	_____	28. rheumat/o	_____
13. nephr/o	_____	29. rhin/o	_____
14. neur/o	_____	30. thorac/o	_____
15. nos/o	_____	31. ur/o	_____
16. obstetr/o	_____	32. vascul/o	_____

SUFFIXES

Suffix	Meaning	Suffix	Meaning
1. -algia	_____	9. -megaly	_____
2. -ary	_____	10. -oma	_____
3. -cele	_____	11. -osis	_____
4. -eal	_____	12. -rrhea	_____
5. -genic	_____	13. -scopy	_____
6. -ist	_____	14. -stomy	_____
7. -itis	_____	15. -therapy	_____
8. -logy	_____	16. tomy	_____

COMBINING FORMS

ANSWER KEY ➤

1. heart	17. tumor
2. colon	18. eye
3. skin	19. eye
4. endocrine glands	20. straight
5. intestines	21. ear
6. sensation	22. disease
7. stomach	23. child
8. old age	24. mind
9. woman	25. lung
10. blood	26. x-rays
11. treatment	27. rectum
12. voice box	28. flow, fluid
13. kidney	29. nose
14. nerve	30. chest
15. disease	31. urinary tract
16. midwife	32. blood vessels

SUFFIXES

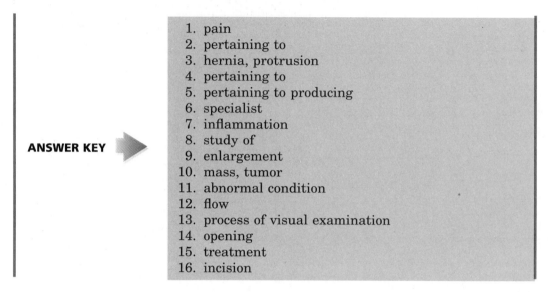

ANSWER KEY

1. pain
2. pertaining to
3. hernia, protrusion
4. pertaining to
5. pertaining to producing
6. specialist
7. inflammation
8. study of
9. enlargement
10. mass, tumor
11. abnormal condition
12. flow
13. process of visual examination
14. opening
15. treatment
16. incision

VII. Pronunciation of Terms

The terms that you have learned in this chapter are presented here with their pronunciations. The capitalized letters in boldface are the accented syllable. Pronounce each word out loud, then write the meaning in the space provided.

Term	Pronunciation	Meaning
anesthesiology	an-es-the-ze-**OL**-o-je	
cardiologist	kar-de-**OL**-o-jist	
cardiovascular surgeon	kar-de-o-**VAS**-ku-lar **SUR**-jin	
clinical	**KLIN**-eh-kal	
colorectal surgeon	ko-lo-**REK**-tal **SUR**-jin	
colostomy	ko-**LOS**-to-me	

dermatologist	der-mah-**TOL**-o-jist _____
dermatology	der-mah-**TOL**-o-je _____
emergency medicine	e-**MER**-jen-se **MED**-ih-sin _____
endocrinologist	en-do-krih-**NOL**-o-jist _____
enteritis	en-teh-**RI**-tis _____
family practice	**FAM**-ih-le **PRAK**-tis _____
gastroenterologist	gas-tro-en-ter-**OL**-o-jist _____
gastroscopy	gas-**TROS**-ko-pe _____
geriatric	jer-e-**AH**-trik _____
geriatrician	jer-e-ah-**TRISH**-shun _____
gynecologist	gi-neh-**KOL**-o-jist _____
gynecology	gi-neh-**KOL**-o-je _____
hematologist	he-mah-**TOL**-o-jist _____
hematoma	he-mah-**TO**-mah _____
iatrogenic	i-ah-tro-**JEN**-ik _____
infectious disease	in-**FEK**-shus dih-**ZEZ** _____
internal medicine	in-**TER**-nal **MED**-ih-sin _____
laryngitis	lah-rin-**JI**-tis _____

nephrologist	neh-**FROL**-o-jist
nephrostomy	neh-**FROS**-to-me
neuralgia	nu-**RAL**-je-ah
neurologist	nu-**ROL**-o-jist
neurosurgeon	nu-ro-**SUR**-jin
nosocomial	no-zo-**KO**-me-al
obstetrician	ob-steh-**TRISH**-un
obstetrics	ob-**STET**-riks
oncogenic	ong-ko-**JEN**-ik
oncologist	ong-**KOL**-o-jist
ophthalmologist	of-thal-**MOL**-o-jist
ophthalmology	of-thal-**MOL**-o-je
optician	op-**TISH**-un
optometrist	op-**TOM**-eh-trist
orthopedist	orth-o-**PE**-dist
otitis	o-**TI**-tis
otolaryngologist	o-to-lar-in-**GOL**-o-jist
pathologist	pah-**THOL**-o-jist

pathology	pah-**THOL**-o-je
pediatric	pe-de-**AT**-rik
pediatrician	pe-de-ah-**TRISH**-un
psychiatrist	si-**KI**-ah-trist
psychosis	si-**KO**-sis
pulmonary specialist	**PUL**-mo-ner-e **SPESH**-ah-list
radiologist	ra-de-**OL**-o-jist
radiation oncologist	ra-de-**A**-shun ong-**KOL**-o-jist
radiotherapy	ra-de-o-**THER**-ah-pe
rectocele	**REK**-to-sel
research	**RE**-surch
rheumatologist	ru-mah-**TOL**-o-jist
rheumatology	ru-mah-**TOL**-o-je
rhinorrhea	ri-no-**RE**-ah
surgery	**SIR**-jer-e
thoracic surgeon	tho-**RAS**-ik **SUR**-jin
thoracotomy	tho-rah-**KOT**-o-me
urologist	u-**ROL**-o-jist
vasculitis	vas-ku-**LI**-tis

VIII. Practical Applications

The following are three groups of allied health specialists. Match each specialist with a job description below:

Group A

1. anesthesiologist assistant   _____

2. audiologist   _____

3. blood bank technologist   _____

4. chiropractor   _____

5. clinical laboratory technician   _____

6. dental assistant   _____

7. dental hygenist   _____

8. dental laboratory technician   _____

9. diagnostic medical sonographer   _____

10. dietitian/nutritionist   _____

a) Treats patients with health problems associated with the muscular, nervous, and skeletal systems, especially the spine
b) Prepares materials (crowns, bridges) for use by a dentist
c) Works with people who have hearing problems by using testing devices to measure hearing loss
d) Provides preventive dental care and teaches the practice of good oral hygiene
e) Collects, types, and prepares blood and its components for transfusions
f) Aids in the delivery of anesthesia during surgery
g) Assists a dentist with dental procedures
h) Performs diagnostic ultrasound procedures
i) Plans nutrition programs and supervises the preparation and serving of meals
j) Performs tests to examine and analyze body fluids, tissues, and cells

Group B

1.   EKG technician   _____

2.   emergency medical technician/paramedic   _____

3.   health information administrator   _____

4.   home health aide   _____

5.   licensed practical nurse   _____

6.   medical assistant   _____

7.   medical laboratory technician   _____

8.   nuclear medicine technologist   _____

9.   nursing aide   _____

10. occupational therapist   _____

a) Cares for elderly, disabled, and ill persons in their own homes, helping them live there instead of in an institution
b) Performs routine tests and laboratory procedures
c) Manages, plans, organizes, supervises, and evaluates institutional and community resources involving the needs and demands of health care
d) Operates an electrocardiograph to record EKGs, Holter monitoring, and stress tests
e) Performs radioactive tests and procedures under the supervision of a nuclear medicine physician, who interprets the results
f) Gives immediate care and transports sick or injured to medical facilities
g) Helps physicians examine and treat patients and performs tasks to keep offices running smoothly
h) Cares for the sick, injured, convalescing, and handicapped, under the direct supervision of physicians and registered nurses; provides basic bedside care

(*Continued*)

i) Helps individuals with mentally, physically, developmentally, emotionally disabling conditions to develop, recover, or maintain daily living and working skills

j) Helps care for physically or mentally ill, injured or disabled patients confined to nursing, hospital, or residential care facilities; known as nursing assistants or hospital attendants

Group C

1. ophthalmic medical technician ＿＿＿＿

2. phlebotomist ＿＿＿＿

3. physical therapist ＿＿＿＿

4. physician assistant ＿＿＿＿

5. radiation therapy technician ＿＿＿＿

6. radiographer/radiological technician ＿＿＿＿

7. registered nurse ＿＿＿＿

8. respiratory therapist ＿＿＿＿

9. speech language pathologist ＿＿＿＿

10. surgical technologist ＿＿＿＿

a) Evaluates, treats, and cares for patients with breathing disorders

b) Draws and tests blood under the supervision of a medical technologist or laboratory manager

c) Cares for sick and injured people by assessing and recording symptoms, assisting physicians during treatments and examinations, and administering medications

d) Prepares cancer patients for treatment and administers prescribed doses of ionizing radiation to specific areas of the body

e) Helps ophthalmologists provide medical eye care

f) Examines, diagnoses, and treats patients, under the direct supervision of a physician

g) Assists in operations under the supervision of surgeons or registered nurses

h) Improves the mobility, relieves the pain, and prevents or limits permanent physical disabilities of patients suffering from injuries or disease

i) Produces x-ray images of parts of the body for use in diagnosing medical problems

j) Assesses and treats persons with speech, language, voice, and fluency disorders

ANSWER KEY ➤

Group A
| 1. f | 2. c | 3. e | 4. a | 5. j |
| 6. g | 7. d | 8. b | 9. h | 10. i |

Group B
| 1. d | 2. f | 3. c | 4. a | 5. h |
| 6. g | 7. b | 8. e | 9. j | 10. i |

Group C
| 1. e | 2. b | 3. h | 4. f | 5. d |
| 6. i | 7. c | 8. a | 9. j | 10. g |

Body Systems

This appendix contains four-color diagrams of body systems. Major organs and structures are labeled for your reference, and definitions for these parts of the body are listed in the *Glossary of Medical Terms* on page 241. Combining forms for parts of the body are given in parentheses next to each label on the diagram. For easy reference, these combining forms are also listed in the *Glossary of Word Parts* on page 273. This information will help you analyze medical terms as you work through the text.

On the page following each body systems diagram, you will find a list of combining forms and examples of terminology utilizing each word part. In addition, this page contains a short list and explanations of pathological conditions commonly associated with each system of the body. Hopefully, this can be a focus of study in your classes, and also be useful as a reference for your work in the medical field.

I. Cardiovascular System
II. Digestive System
III. Endocrine System*
IV. Female Reproductive System*
V. Lymphatic System*
VI. Male Reproductive System*

VII. Musculoskeletal System*
VIII. Nervous System†
IX. Respiratory System*
X. Skin and Sense Organs*
XI. Urinary System*

---

*Figures adapted from Chabner DE: The Language of Medicine. 5th edition. Philadelphia, WB Saunders Co, 1996.
†Figure adapted from Fowler I: Human Anatomy. Belmont, CA, Wadsworth Publishing, 1984.

ANATOMY

Circulation of Blood

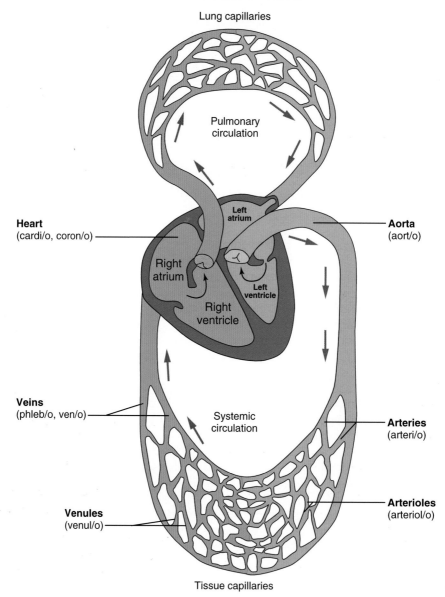

Colored vessels contain blood that is rich in oxygen. Arrows show the path of blood flow from the tissue capillaries through venules and veins toward the heart, to the lung capillaries, back to the heart, out the aorta to the arteries and arterioles, and then to the tissue capillaries.

TERMINOLOGY

Meanings for terminology are found in the *Glossary of Medical Terms*.

Combining Form	Meaning	Terminology	Meaning
angi/o	vessel	angioplasty	
aort/o	aorta	aortic stenosis	
arteri/o	artery	arteriosclerosis	
arteriol/o	arteriole	arteriolitis	
cardi/o	heart	cardiomyopathy	
coron/o	heart	coronary arteries	
phleb/o	vein	phlebotomy	
ven/o	vein	intravenous	
venul/o	venule	venulitis	

PATHOLOGY

Definitions for terminology in boldface are found in the *Glossary of Medical Terms*.

Angina pectoris: Chest pain caused by decreased blood flow to heart muscle.

Aneurysm: Local widening of an artery caused by weakness in the arterial wall or breakdown of the wall owing to atherosclerosis.

Arrhythmia: Abnormal heart beat (rhythm)—**fibrillation** and **flutter** are examples.

Atherosclerosis: Hardening of arteries with a collection of cholesterol-like plaque.

Congestive heart failure: Inability of the heart to pump its required amount of blood. Blood accumulates in the lungs causing **pulmonary edema**.

Hypertension: High blood pressure. **Essential hypertension** is high blood pressure with no apparent cause. In **secondary hypertension**, another illness (kidney disease, or adrenal gland disorder) is the cause of the high blood pressure.

Myocardial infarction: Heart attack. An **infarction** is an area of dead (**necrotic**) tissue.

Shock: A group of symptoms (paleness of skin, weak and rapid pulse, shallow breathing) that indicate poor oxygen supply to tissues and insufficient return of blood to the heart.

ANATOMY

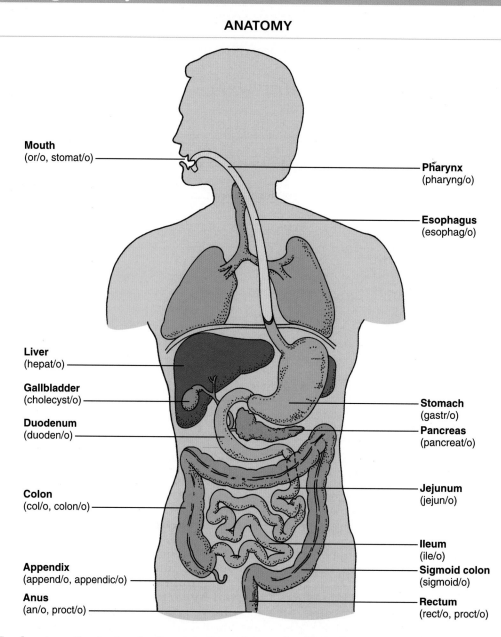

Mouth
(or/o, stomat/o)

Pharynx
(pharyng/o)

Esophagus
(esophag/o)

Liver
(hepat/o)

Gallbladder
(cholecyst/o)

Duodenum
(duoden/o)

Stomach
(gastr/o)

Pancreas
(pancreat/o)

Colon
(col/o, colon/o)

Jejunum
(jejun/o)

Ileum
(ile/o)

Appendix
(append/o, appendic/o)

Sigmoid colon
(sigmoid/o)

Anus
(an/o, proct/o)

Rectum
(rect/o, proct/o)

Food enters the body via the mouth and travels through the pharynx, esophagus, and stomach to the small intestine. The liver, gallbladder, and pancreas make and store chemicals that aid in the digestion of foods. Digested (broken down) food is absorbed into the bloodstream through the walls of the small intestine. Any food that cannot be absorbed continues into the colon (large intestine) and leaves the body through the rectum and anus.

TERMINOLOGY

Combining Form	Meaning	Terminology	Meaning
cholecyst/o	gallbladder	cholecystectomy	_removal of cyst of gallbladder_
col/o colon/o	colon	colostomy	_cutting into the colon_
		colonoscopy	_process of viewing colon_
duoden/o	duodenum	duodenal	_pertains to duodenum_
esophag/o	esophagus	esophageal	_pertaining to esophagus_
gastr/o	stomach	gastralgia	_pain in the stomach_
hepat/o	liver	hepatomegaly	_enlargement of liver_
ile/o	ileum	ileostomy	_to cut into ileum_
jejun/o	jejunum	gastrojejunostomy	_to cut into jejunum_
or/o	mouth	oral	_pertaining to the mouth_
pancreat/o	pancreas	pancreatitis	_inflammation of the pancreas_
pharyng/o	pharynx	pharyngeal	_pharynx_
proct/o	anus and rectum	proctoscopy	_to view anus and rectum with instrument_
stomat/o	mouth	stomatitis	_inflammation of mouth_

PATHOLOGY

Cholelithiasis: Abnormal condition of gallstones.

Cirrhosis: Chronic disease of the liver with degeneration of liver cells.

Colonic polyposis: **Polyps** (small growths) protrude from the mucous membrane lining the colon.

Diverticulosis: Abnormal condition of small pouches or sacs (**diverticula**) in the wall of the intestine (often the colon).

Hepatitis: Inflammation of the liver.

Inflammatory bowel disease: Inflammation of the terminal (last) portion of the ileum (**Crohn disease**) or inflammation of the colon (**ulcerative colitis**).

Jaundice: Yellow-orange coloration of the skin and other tissues.

ANATOMY

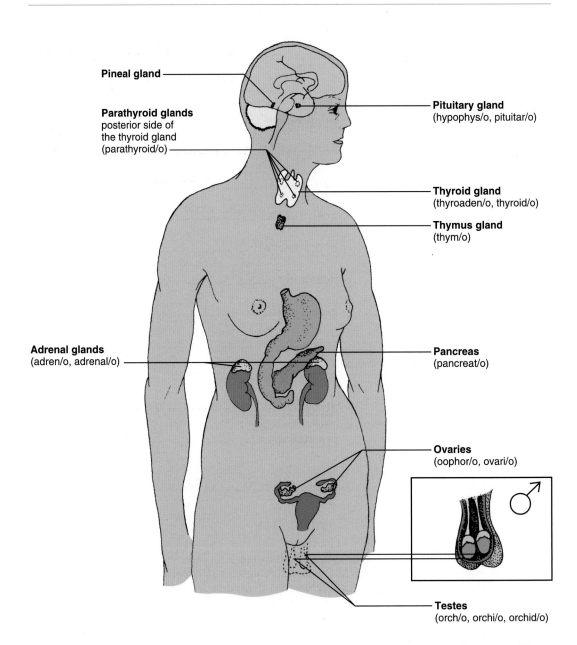

Pineal gland

Parathyroid glands
posterior side of
the thyroid gland
(parathyroid/o)

Pituitary gland
(hypophys/o, pituitar/o)

Thyroid gland
(thyroaden/o, thyroid/o)

Thymus gland
(thym/o)

Adrenal glands
(adren/o, adrenal/o)

Pancreas
(pancreat/o)

Ovaries
(oophor/o, ovari/o)

Testes
(orch/o, orchi/o, orchid/o)

Endocrine glands secrete (form and give off) hormones into the bloodstream. The hormones travel throughout the body and affect organs (including other endocrine glands) to control their actions.

TERMINOLOGY

Combining Form	Meaning	Terminology	Meaning
adren/o adrenal/o	adrenal gland	adrenopathy	_gland pathology_
		adrenalectomy	
hypophys/o	pituitary gland	hypophyseal	_pertaining to pituitary gland_
oophor/o ovari/o	ovary	oophoritis	_inflammation of ovaries_
		ovarian cyst	_ovarian_
orch/o orchi/o orchid/o	testis	orchitis	
		orchiopexy	
		orchidectomy	
pancreat/o	pancreas	pancreatectomy	
parathyroid/o	parathyroid gland	hyperparathyroidism	
pituitar/o	pituitary gland	hypopituitarism	
thym/o	thymus gland	thymoma	
thyroaden/o thyroid/o	thyroid gland	thyroadenitis	
		thyroidectomy	

PATHOLOGY

Acromegaly: Enlargement of extremities caused by hypersecretion of the anterior portion of the pituitary gland after puberty.

Cushing syndrome: A group of symptoms produced by excess secretion of **cortisol** from the **adrenal cortex**. These symptoms include obesity, moon-like fullness of the face, hyperglycemia, and **osteoporosis**.

Diabetes mellitus: A disorder of the pancreas that causes increase in blood sugar. **Type I diabetes**, with onset usually in childhood, involves complete deficiency of **insulin** in the body. **Type II diabetes**, with onset usually in adulthood, involves some insulin deficiency and resistance of tissues to the action of insulin.

Goiter: Enlargement of the thyroid gland.

Hyperthyroidism: Overactivity of the thyroid gland; also called **Graves disease** or **exophthalmic** (eyeballs bulge outward) **goiter**.

193

ANATOMY

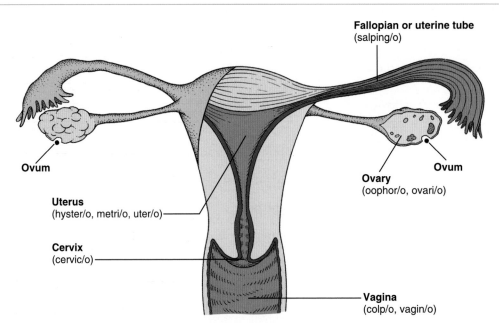

An egg cell (ovum) is produced in the ovary and travels through the uterine (fallopian) tube. If a sperm cell is present and fertilization (the union of the egg and sperm cell) takes place, the resulting cell (embryo) may implant in the lining of the uterus. The embryo (later called the fetus) develops in the uterus for nine months and is delivered from the body through the cervix and vagina.

TERMINOLOGY

Combining Form	Meaning	Terminology	Meaning
cervic/o	cervix	cervical _____	
colp/o vagin/o	vagina	colposcopy _____	
		vaginitis _____	
hyster/o metri/o uter/o	uterus	hysterectomy _____	
		endometrium _____	
		uterine _____	
oophor/o ovari/o	ovary	oophorectomy _____	
		ovarian cancer _____	
salping/o	fallopian tube	salpingectomy _____	

PATHOLOGY

Amenorrhea: Absence of menstrual flow.

Dysmenorrhea: Painful menstrual flow.

Endometriosis: Tissue from the inner lining of the uterus (endometrium) occurs abnormally in other pelvic or abdominal locations (fallopian tubes, ovaries, or peritoneum).

Ectopic pregnancy: Pregnancy that is not in the uterus; usually occurring in a fallopian tube.

Fibroids: Benign tumors in the uterus. A fibroid is also called a **leiomyoma** (tumor of smooth or involuntary muscle). Lei/o means smooth.

Menorrhagia: Excessive discharge (-rrhagia) of blood from the uterus during menstruation.

Pelvic inflammatory disease: Inflammation (often caused by bacterial infection) in the region of the pelvis. Because the condition primarily affects the fallopian tubes, it is also called **salpingitis**.

ANATOMY

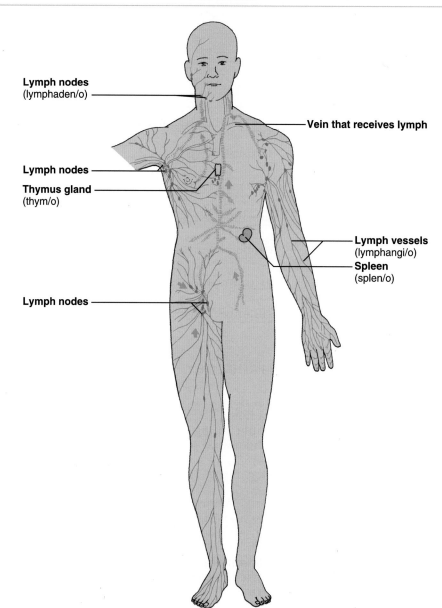

Lymph nodes
(lymphaden/o)

Vein that receives lymph

Lymph nodes

Thymus gland
(thym/o)

Lymph vessels
(lymphangi/o)

Spleen
(splen/o)

Lymph nodes

Lymph originates in the tissue spaces around cells, travels in lymph vessels and through lymph nodes to a large vein in the neck where it enters the bloodstream. Lymph contains white blood cells (lymphocytes) that help the body fight disease. The spleen produces lymphocytes and disposes of dying blood cells. The thymus gland also produces lymphocytes.

196

TERMINOLOGY

Combining Form	Meaning	Terminology	Meaning
lymph/o	lymph fluid	lymphopoiesis _____	
lymphaden/o	lymph node ("gland")	lymphadenectomy _____	
		lymphadenopathy _____	
lymphangi/o	lymph vessel	lymphangiography _____	
splen/o	spleen	splenomegaly _____	
thym/o	thymus gland	thymoma _____	

PATHOLOGY

Acquired immunodeficiency syndrome (AIDS): Suppression or deficiency of the immune response (destruction of lymphocytes) caused by exposure to **HIV (human immunodeficiency virus)**.

Lymphoma: Malignant tumor of lymph nodes and lymphatic tissue. **Hodgkin disease** is an example of a lymphoma.

Mononucleosis: Acute infectious disease with enlargement of lymph nodes and increased numbers of **lymphocytes** and **monocytes** (white blood cells) in the bloodstream.

Sarcoidosis: Inflammatory disease in which small nodules, or tubercles, form in lymph nodes and other organs. Sarc/o is flesh and -oid means resembling.

ANATOMY

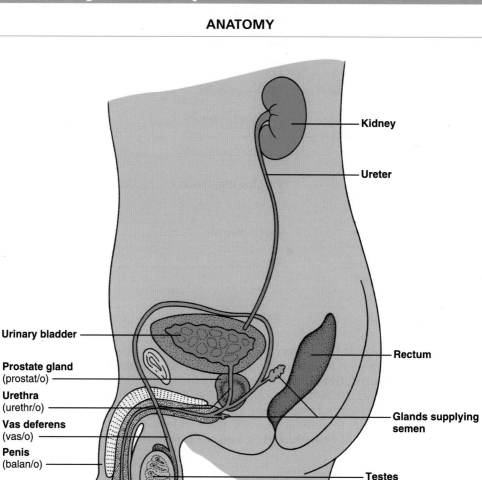

Kidney

Ureter

Urinary bladder

Prostate gland
(prostat/o)

Urethra
(urethr/o)

Vas deferens
(vas/o)

Penis
(balan/o)

Rectum

Glands supplying
semen

Testes
(orch/o, orchi/o, orchid/o)

Scrotum
(scrot/o)

Sperm cells are produced in the testes (singular: testis) and travel up into the body, through the vas deferens, and around the urinary bladder. The vas deferens unites with the urethra, which opens to the outside of the body through the penis. The prostate and the other glands near the urethra produce a fluid (semen) that leaves the body with sperm cells.

TERMINOLOGY

Combining Form	Meaning	Terminology	Meaning
balan/o	penis	balanitis _____	
orch/o orchi/o orchid/o	testis	orchitis _____	
		orchiectomy _____	
		orchidectomy _____	
prostat/o	prostate gland	prostatectomy _____	
scrot/o	scrotum	scrotal _____	
urethr/o	urethra	urethritis _____	
vas/o	vas deferens	vasectomy _____	

PATHOLOGY

Benign prostatic hyperplasia: Noncancerous enlargement of the prostate gland.

Cryptorchidism: Condition of undescended testis. The testis is not in the scrotal sac at birth. Crypt/o means hidden.

Hydrocele: Sac of clear fluid in the scrotum. Hydr/o means water and -cele is a hernia (a bulging or swelling).

Prostatic carcinoma: Cancer of the prostate gland.

Testicular carcinoma: Malignant tumor of the testis. An example is a **seminoma**.

Variocele: Enlarged, swollen veins near a testicle. Varic/o means swollen veins.

ANATOMY

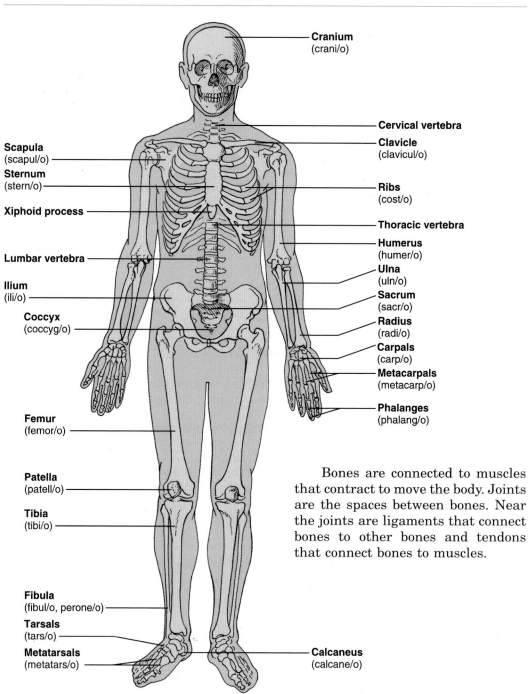

Scapula
(scapul/o)

Sternum
(stern/o)

Xiphoid process

Lumbar vertebra

Ilium
(ili/o)

Coccyx
(coccyg/o)

Femur
(femor/o)

Patella
(patell/o)

Tibia
(tibi/o)

Fibula
(fibul/o, perone/o)

Tarsals
(tars/o)

Metatarsals
(metatars/o)

Cranium
(crani/o)

Cervical vertebra

Clavicle
(clavicul/o)

Ribs
(cost/o)

Thoracic vertebra

Humerus
(humer/o)

Ulna
(uln/o)

Sacrum
(sacr/o)

Radius
(radi/o)

Carpals
(carp/o)

Metacarpals
(metacarp/o)

Phalanges
(phalang/o)

Calcaneus
(calcane/o)

Bones are connected to muscles that contract to move the body. Joints are the spaces between bones. Near the joints are ligaments that connect bones to other bones and tendons that connect bones to muscles.

TERMINOLOGY

Combining Form	Meaning	Terminology	Meaning
arthr/o	joint	arthroscopy _____	
chondr/o	cartilage	chondroma _____	
cost/o	rib	costochondritis _____	
crani/o	skull	craniotomy _____	
ligament/o	ligament	ligamentous _____	
my/o myos/o muscul/o	muscle	myosarcoma _____	
		myositis _____	
		muscular _____	
myel/o	bone marrow	myelodysplasia _____	
oste/o	bone	osteomyelitis _____	
pelv/o	pelvis, hipbone	pelvic _____	
spondyl/o vertebr/o	vertebra	spondylosis _____	
		intervertebral _____	
ten/o tendin/o	tendon	tenorrhaphy _____	
		tendinitis _____	

PATHOLOGY

Ankylosing spondylitis: Chronic, progressive arthritis with stiffening (**ankylosis**) of joints, primarily of the spine and hip.

Carpal tunnel syndrome: Compression of the median nerve as it passes between the ligament and the bones and tendons of the wrist.

Gouty arthritis: Inflammation of joints caused by excessive uric acid; **gout**.

Muscular dystrophy: An inherited disorder characterized by progressive weakness and degeneration of muscle fibers.

Osteoporosis: Decrease in bone density with thinning and weakening of bone. Porosis means containing passages or spaces.

Rheumatoid arthritis: Chronic inflammation of joints; pain, swelling and stiffening, especially in the small joints of the hands and feet. Rheum- means a "flowing," descriptive of the swelling in joints.

ANATOMY

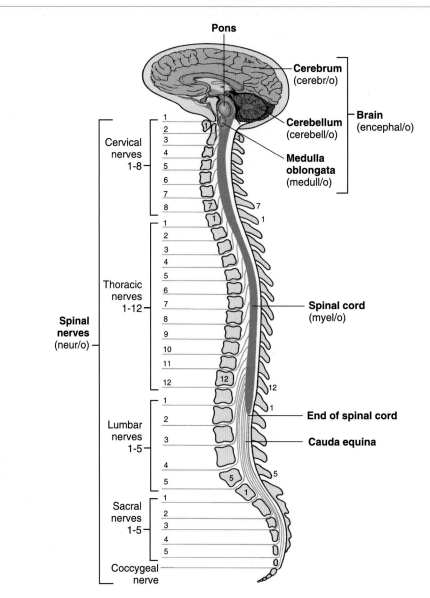

Pons

Cerebrum
(cerebr/o)

Cerebellum
(cerebell/o)

Brain
(encephal/o)

Medulla
oblongata
(medull/o)

Cervical
nerves
1-8

1
2
3
4
5
6
7
8

Thoracic
nerves
1-12

1
2
3
4
5
6
7
8
9
10
11
12

Spinal
nerves
(neur/o)

Spinal cord
(myel/o)

Lumbar
nerves
1-5

1
2
3
4
5

End of spinal cord

Cauda equina

Sacral
nerves
1-5

1
2
3
4
5

Coccygeal
nerve

The central nervous system is the brain and the spinal cord. The peripheral nervous system includes the nerves that carry messages to and from the brain and spinal cord. Spinal nerves carry messages to and from the spinal cord, and the cranial nerves (not pictured) carry messages to and from the brain.

Combining Form	Meaning	Terminology	Meaning
cerebell/o	cerebellum	cerebellar _____	
cerebr/o	cerebrum	cerebral _____	
encephal/o	brain	encephalitis _____	
medull/o	medulla oblongata	medullary _____	
myel/o	spinal cord	myelography _____	
neur/o	nerve	neuropathy _____	

PATHOLOGY

Alzheimer disease: Brain disorder marked by deterioration of mental capacity (**dementia**).

Cerebrovascular accident: Damage to the blood vessels of the cerebrum, leading to loss of blood supply to brain tissue; a **stroke**.

Concussion: Brief loss of consciousness due to injury to the brain.

Epilepsy: Chronic brain disorder characterized by recurrent seizure activity.

Glioblastoma: Malignant brain tumor arising from **neuroglial** (supportive and connective tissue in the brain) cells. Blast- means immature.

Hemiplegia: **Paralysis** (-plegia) that affects the right or left half of the body.

Meningitis: Inflammation of the **meninges** (membranes surrounding the brain and spinal cord).

Multiple sclerosis: Destruction of the **myelin sheath** on nerve cells in the central nervous system (brain and spinal cord), with replacement by plaques of sclerotic (hard) tissue.

Paraplegia: Paralysis that affects the lower portion of the body. From the Greek meaning to strike (-plegia) on one side (para-). This term was previously used to describe hemiplegia.

Syncope: Fainting; sudden and temporary loss of consciousness due to inadequate flow of blood to the brain.

ANATOMY

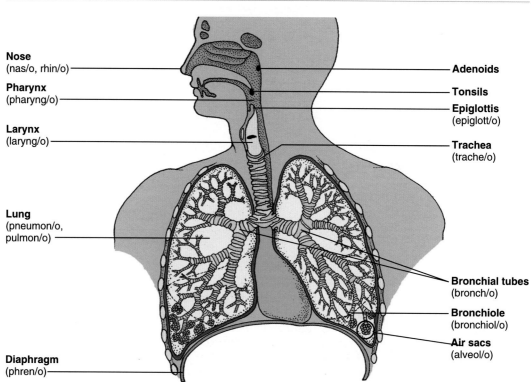

Nose
(nas/o, rhin/o)

Pharynx
(pharyng/o)

Larynx
(laryng/o)

Lung
(pneumon/o,
pulmon/o)

Diaphragm
(phren/o)

Adenoids

Tonsils

Epiglottis
(epiglott/o)

Trachea
(trache/o)

Bronchial tubes
(bronch/o)

Bronchiole
(bronchiol/o)

Air sacs
(alveol/o)

Air enters the nose and travels to the pharynx (throat). From the pharynx, air passes the epiglottis and larynx (voice box) into the trachea (windpipe). The trachea splits into two tubes, the bronchial tubes, that carry air into the lungs. The bronchial tubes divide into smaller tubes called bronchioles that end in small air sacs. Thin air sacs allow oxygen to pass through them into tiny capillaries containing red blood cells. Red blood cells transport the oxygen to all parts of the body.

In a similar manner, gaseous waste (carbon dioxide) leaves the blood to enter air sacs and then travels out of the body through bronchioles, bronchial tubes, trachea, larynx, pharynx, and the nose.

TERMINOLOGY

Combining Form	Meaning	Terminology	Meaning
alveol/o	air sac; alveolus	alveolar _____	
bronch/o	bronchial tube	bronchoscopy _____	
bronchiol/o	bronchiole	bronchiolitis _____	
epiglott/o	epiglottis	epiglottitis _____	
laryng/o	larynx	laryngeal _____	
nas/o rhin/o	nose	nasal _____	
		rhinorrhea _____	
pharyng/o	pharynx	pharyngitis _____	
phren/o	diaphragm	phrenic _____	
pneumon/o pulmon/o	lung	pneumonectomy _____	
		pulmonary _____	
trache/o	trachea	tracheostomy _____	

PATHOLOGY

Asphyxia: Extreme decrease in the amount of **oxygen** in the body with increase of **carbon dioxide** leads to loss of consciousness or death.

Asthma: Spasm and narrowing of bronchi leading to bronchial airway obstruction.

Atelectasis: Collapsed lung (atel/o means incomplete and -ectasis is dilation or expansion).

Emphysema: Hyperinflation of air sacs with destruction of alveolar walls. Along with chronic bronchitis and asthma, emphysema is a type of **chronic obstructive pulmonary disease**.

Hemoptysis: Spitting up of blood.

Hemothorax: Blood in the pleural cavity (space between the **pleura**).

Pneumonia: Inflammation and infection of alveoli, which fill with pus or products of the inflammatory reaction.

Pneumoconiosis: Abnormal condition of dust (coni/o) in the lungs.

Tuberculosis: An infectious disease caused by bacteria (**bacilli**). Lungs are affected and other organs as well. Symptoms are cough, weight loss, night sweats, hemoptysis (spitting up blood), and pleuritic pain.

ANATOMY

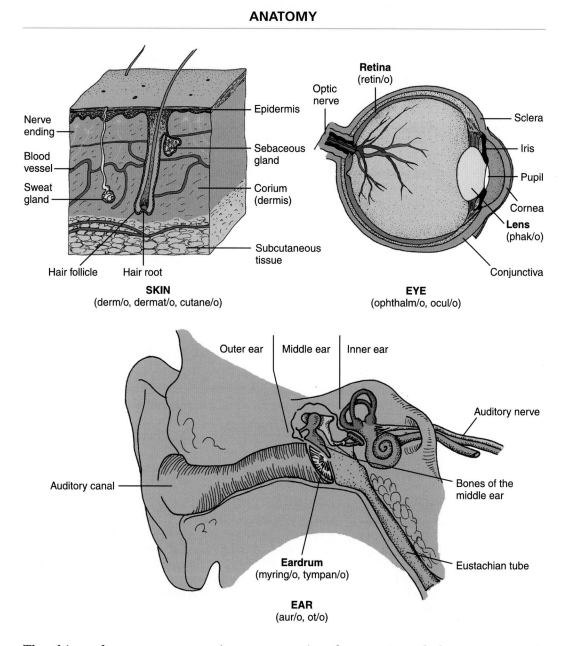

SKIN
(derm/o, dermat/o, cutane/o)

Labels: Nerve ending, Blood vessel, Sweat gland, Hair follicle, Hair root, Epidermis, Sebaceous gland, Corium (dermis), Subcutaneous tissue

EYE
(ophthalm/o, ocul/o)

Labels: Retina (retin/o), Optic nerve, Sclera, Iris, Pupil, Cornea, Lens (phak/o), Conjunctiva

EAR
(aur/o, ot/o)

Labels: Outer ear, Middle ear, Inner ear, Auditory nerve, Auditory canal, Bones of the middle ear, Eardrum (myring/o, tympan/o), Eustachian tube

The skin and sense organs receive messages (touch sensations, light waves, sound waves) from the environment and send them to the brain via nerves. These messages are interpreted in the brain, making sight, hearing, and perception of the environment possible.

206

TERMINOLOGY

Combining Form	Meaning	Terminology	Meaning
aur/o ot/o	ear	aural discharge _____	
		otitis _____	
cutane/o derm/o dermat/o	skin	subcutaneous _____	
		epidermis _____	
		dermatology _____	
myring/o tympan/o	eardrum	myringtomy _____	
		tympanoplasty _____	
ocul/o ophthalm/o	eye	ocular _____	
		ophthalmoscope _____	
phak/o	lens of the eye	aphakia _____	
retin/o	retina	retinopathy _____	

PATHOLOGY

Alopecia: Absence of hair from areas where it normally grows; baldness.

Cataract: Clouding (opacity) of the lens of the eye, causing impairment of vision or blindness.

Conjunctivitis: Inflammation of the **conjunctiva** (mucous membrane lining the inner surface of the eyelid and exposed surface of the eyeball).

Glaucoma: Increase in pressure (fluid accumulation) within the chamber at the front of the eye.

Melanoma: Malignant tumor of pigmented cells (melan/o means black) that arises from a **nevus** (mole) in the skin.

Nevus: Pigmented lesion in or on the skin; a mole.

Tinnitus: Abnormal noise (ringing, buzzing, roaring) sound in the ears.

ANATOMY

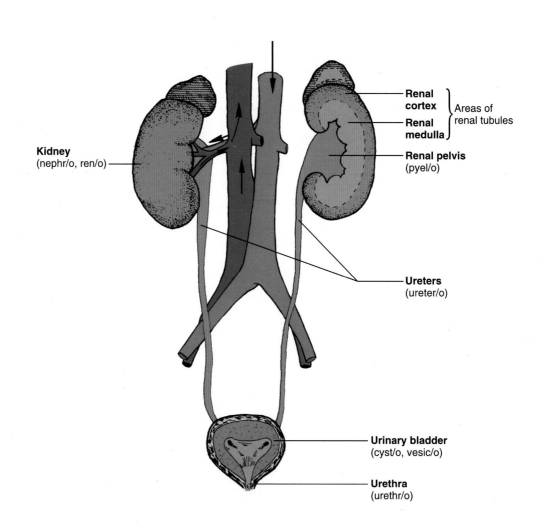

Kidney
(nephr/o, ren/o)

Renal cortex
Renal medulla
} Areas of renal tubules

Renal pelvis
(pyel/o)

Ureters
(ureter/o)

Urinary bladder
(cyst/o, vesic/o)

Urethra
(urethr/o)

Urine is formed as waste materials, such as urea, are filtered from the blood into the tubules of the kidney. Urine passes from the tubules into the central collecting section of the kidney, the renal pelvis. Each renal pelvis leads directly to a ureter, which takes the urine to the urinary bladder. The bladder releases urine to the urethra and urine leaves the body.

TERMINOLOGY

Combining Form	Meaning	Terminology	Meaning
cyst/o vesic/o	urinary bladder	cystoscopy _____	
		vesical _____	
nephr/o ren/o	kidney	nephritis _____	
		renal _____	
pyel/o	renal pelvis	pyelogram _____	
ureter/o	ureter	ureterectomy _____	
urethr/o	urethra	urethritis _____	

PATHOLOGY

Albuminuria: Abnormal condition of protein (albumin) in the urine.
Anuria: Abnormal condition of no urine production.
Dysuria: Painful urination.
Glycosuria: Abnormal condition of sugar in the urine.
Hematuria: Abnormal condition of blood in the urine.
Nephrolithiasis: Abnormal condition of stones in the kidney.
Renal failure: Kidneys stop functioning and do not produce urine.
Uremia: Condition of high levels of **urea** (nitrogenous waste material) in the blood.

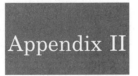

Appendix II

Diagnostic Tests and Procedures

RADIOLOGY, ULTRASOUND, AND IMAGING PROCEDURES

In many of the following procedures a *contrast* substance (sometimes referred to as a *dye*) is introduced into or around a body part so that the part can be viewed while x-rays are taken. The contrast substance (often containing barium or iodine) appears dense on the x-ray and outlines the body part that it fills.

The suffix -GRAPY, meaning "process of recording," is used in many terms describing imaging procedures. The suffix -GRAM, meaning "record," is also used and describes the actual image that is produced by the procedure.

Pronunciation of each term is given with its meaning. The syllable that gets the accent is in **CAPITAL LETTERS**. Terms in SMALL CAPITAL LETTERS are defined elsewhere in the appendix.

ANGIOGRAPHY (an-je-OG-rah-fe) or ANGIOGRAM (AN-je-o-gram): X-ray recording of blood vessels. A contrast substance is injected into blood vessels (veins and arteries), and x-ray pictures are taken of the vessels. In *cerebral angiography*, x-ray pictures are taken of blood vessels in the brain. Angiography is used to detect abnormalities in blood vessels, such as blockage, malformation, and arteriosclerosis. Angiography is performed most frequently to view arteries and is often used interchangeably with *arteriography*.

ARTERIOGRAPHY (ar-ter-e-OG-rah-fe) or ARTERIOGRAM (ar-TER-e-oh-gram): X-ray recording of arteries after injection of a contrast substance into an artery. *Coronary arteriography* is the visualization of arteries that bring blood to the heart muscle.

BARIUM TESTS (BAR-re-um tests): X-ray examinations using a liquid barium mixture to locate disorders in the esophagus (*esophagogram*), duodenum, small intestine (*small bowel follow through*), and colon (*barium enema*). Taken before or during the examination, barium causes the intestinal tract to stand out in silhouette when viewed through a *fluoroscope* or seen on an x-ray film. The *barium swallow* is used to examine the upper gastrointestinal tract, and the *barium enema* is for examination of the lower gastrointestinal tract.

BARIUM ENEMA: See LOWER GASTROINTESTINAL EXAMINATION and BARIUM TESTS.

BARIUM SWALLOW: See ESOPHAGOGRAPHY and BARIUM TESTS.

CARDIAC CATHETERIZATION (KAR-de-ak cath-eh-ter-i-ZA-shun): A catheter (tube) is passed via vein or artery into the chambers of the heart. This procedure is used to measure the blood flow out of the heart and the pressures and oxygen content in the heart chambers. Contrast material is also introduced into heart chambers and x-ray images are taken to show heart structure.

CT SCAN, CAT SCAN: X-ray images are taken to show the body in cross-section. Contrast material may be used (injected into the bloodstream) to highlight structures such as the liver, brain, or blood vessels, and barium can be swallowed to outline gastrointestinal organs. X-ray images, taken as the x-ray tube rotates around the body, are processed by a computer to show "slices" of body tissues, most often within the head, chest, and abdomen.

CEREBRAL ANGIOGRAPHY: See ANGIOGRAPHY.

CHEST X-RAY: An x-ray of the chest may show infection (as in pneumonia or tuberculosis), emphysema, occupational exposure (asbestosis), lung tumors, or heart enlargement.

CHOLANGIOGRAPHY (kol-an-je-OG-rah-fe) or CHOLANGIOGRAM (kol-an-je-o-gram): X-ray recording of bile ducts. Contrast material is given by intravenous injuection (*I.V. cholangiogram*) and collects in the gallbladder and bile ducts or is directly inserted by a tube through the mouth into bile ducts (*T-tube cholangiogram*). X-rays are taken of bile ducts to identify obstructions caused by tumors or stones.

CORONARY ARTERIOGRAPHY: See ARTERIOGRAPHY.

CYSTOGRAPHY (sis-TOG-rah-fe) or CYSTOGRAM (SIS-to-gram): X-ray recording of the urinary bladder using a contrast medium, so that the outline of the urinary bladder can be seen clearly. A contrast substance is injected via catheter into the urethra and urinary bladder, and x-ray images are taken. A *voiding cystourethrogram* is an x-ray image of the urinary tract made while the patient is urinating.

DIGITAL SUBTRACTION ANGIOGRAPHY (DIJ-i-tal sub-TRAK-shun an-je-OG-rah-fe): A unique x-ray technique for viewing blood vessels by taking two images and subtracting one from the other. Images are first taken without contrast and then again after contrast is injected into blood vessels. The first image is then subtracted from the second so that the final image (sharp and precise) shows only contrast-filled blood vessels minus surrounding tissue.

ECHOCARDIOGRAPHY (eh-ko-kar-de-OG-rah-fe) or ECHOCARDIOGRAM (eh-ko-KAR-de-o-gram): Images of the heart are produced by introducing high-frequency sound waves through the chest into the heart. The sound waves are reflected back from the heart, and echoes showing heart structure are displayed on a recording machine. It is a highly useful diagnostic tool in the evaluation of diseases of the valves that separate the heart chambers and diseases of the heart muscle.

ECHOENCEPHALOGRAPHY (eh-ko-en-sef-ah-LOG-rah-fe) or ECHOENCE-PHALOGRAM (eh-ko-en-SEF-ah-lo-gram): An ultrasound recording of the brain. Sound waves are beamed at the brain, and the echoes that return to the machine are recorded as graphic tracings. Brain tumors and hematomas can be detected by abnormal tracings.

ENDOSCOPIC RETROGRADE CHOLANGIOPANCREATOGRAPHY (en-do-SKOP-ik REH-tro-grad kol-an-je-o-pan-kre-ah-TOG-rah-fe): X-ray recording of the bile ducts, pancreas, and pancreatic duct. Contrast is injected via a tube through the mouth into the bile and pancreatic ducts and x-rays are then taken.

ESOPHAGOGRAPHY (eh-sof-ah-GOG-rah-fe) or ESOPHAGOGRAM (eh-SOF-ah-go-gram): Barium sulfate is swallowed and x-ray images are taken of the esophagus. This test is also called a *barium meal* or *barium swallow* and is part of an *upper gastrointestinal examination*.

FLUOROSCOPY (flur-OS-ko-pe): An x-ray procedure that uses a fluorescent screen rather than a photographic plate to show images of the body. X-rays that have passed through the body strike a screen covered with a fluorescent substance that emits yellow-green light. Internal organs are seen directly and in motion. Fluoroscopy is used to guide the insertion of catheters and during *barium tests*.

GALLBLADDER ULTRASOUND (gawl BLA-der UL-tra-sownd): Sound waves are used to visualize gallstones. This procedure has replaced cholecystography, which required ingesting an iodine-based contrast substance.

HYSTEROSALPINGOGRAPHY (his-ter-o-sal-ping-OG-rah-fe) or HYSTERO-SALPINGOGRAM (his-ter-o-sal-PING-o-gram): X-ray recording of the uterus and fallopian tubes. Contrast medium is inserted through the vagina into the uterus and fallopian tubes, and x-rays are taken to detect blockage or tumor.

INTRAVENOUS PYELOGRAPHY: See UROGRAPHY.

LOWER GASTROINTESTINAL EXAMINATION (LO-wer gas-tro-in-TES-tin-al ek-zam-ih-NA-shun): A liquid contrast substance called barium sulfate is inserted through a plastic tube (enema) into the rectum and large intestine (colon). X-ray pictures of the colon are then taken. If tumor is present in the colon, it may appear as an obstruction or irregularity. Also known as a *barium enema*.

LYMPHANGIOGRAPHY (limf-an-je-OG-rah-fe) or LYMPHANGIOGRAM (limf-AN-je-o-gram): X-ray recording of lymph nodes and lymph vessels after contrast is injected into lymphatic vessels in the feet. The contrast medium travels upward through the lymphatic vessels of the pelvis, abdomen, and chest and outlines the architecture of lymph nodes in all areas of the body. This procedure is used to detect tumors within the lymphatic system. It is also known as *lymphography*.

LYMPHOGRAPHY: See LYMPHANGIOGRAPHY.

MAGNETIC RESONANCE IMAGING (mag-NET-ik REZ-o-nans IM-a-jing): Magnetic waves and radiofrequency pulses, not x-rays, are used to create an image of body organs. The images can be taken in several planes of the body—frontal, sagittal (side), and transverse (cross-section)—and are particularly useful for studying brain tumors and tumors of the chest cavity. This procedure is also known as an *MRI*.

MAMMOGRAPHY (mah-MOG-rah-fe) or MAMMOGRAM (MAM-o-gram): X-ray recording of the breast. X-rays of low voltage are beamed at the breast and images are produced. Mammography is used to detect abnormalities in breast tissue, such as early breast cancer.

MYELOGRAPHY (mi-eh-LOG-rah-fe) or MYELOGRAM (MI-eh-lo-gram): X-ray recording of the spinal cord. X-rays are taken of the fluid-filled space surrounding the spinal cord after a contrast medium is injected into the subarachnoid space (between the membranes surrounding the spinal cord) at the lumbar level of the back. Myelography detects tumors or ruptured, "slipped," disks that lie between the backbones (vertebrae) and press on the spinal cord.

PYELOGRAPHY or PYELOGRAM: See UROGRAPHY.

SMALL BOWEL FOLLOW-THROUGH: See BARIUM TESTS and UPPER GASTRO-INTESTINAL EXAMINATION.

TOMOGRAPHY (to-MOG-rah-fe) or TOMOGRAM): X-ray recording that shows an organ in depth. Several pictures ("slices") are taken of an organ by moving the x-ray tube and film in sequence to blur out certain regions and bring others into sharper focus. Tomograms of the kidney and lung are examples.

ULTRASONOGRAPHY (ul-tra-so-NOG-rah-fe) or ULTRASONOGRAM (ul-tra-SON-o-gram): Images are produced by beaming sound waves into the body and capturing the echoes that bounce off organs. These echoes are then processed to produce an image, not in the sharpest detail, but showing the difference between fluid and solid masses and the general position of organs.

UPPER GASTROINTESTINAL EXAMINATION (UP-er gas-tro-in-TES-tin-al ek-zam-ih-NA-shun): A liquid contrast substance called barium sulfate is swallowed and x-ray pictures are taken of the esophagus (*barium meal* or *barium swallow*), duodenum, and small intestine. In a *small bowel follow-through*, pictures are taken at increasing time intervals to follow the progress of barium through the small intestine. Identification of obstructions or ulcers is possible.

UROGRAPHY (u-ROG-rah-fe) or UROGRAM (UR-o-gram): X-ray recording of the kidney and urinary tract. If x-rays are taken after contrast medium is injected intravenously, the procedure is called *intravenous urography* (*descending* or *excretion urography*) or *intravenous pyelography* (*IVP*). If x-rays are taken after injection of contrast medium into the bladder through the urethra, the procedure is *retrograde urography* or *retrograde pyelography*. Pyel/o means renal pelvis (the collecting chamber of the kidney).

NUCLEAR MEDICINE SCANS

In the following diagnostic tests, radioactive material (*radioisotope*) is injected, inhaled, or swallowed and then detected by a scanning device in the organ in which it accumulates. X-rays, ultrasound, or magnetic waves are not used.

Pronunciation of each term is given with its meaning. The syllable that gets the accent is in **CAPITAL LETTERS.**

BONE SCAN: A radioactive substance is injected intravenously, and its uptake in bones is detected by a scanning device. Tumors in bone can be detected by increased uptake of the radioactive material in the areas of the lesions.

BRAIN SCAN: A radioactive substance is injected intravenously and collects in any lesion that disturbs the natural barrier that exists between blood vessels and normal brain tissue (blood-brain barrier), allowing the radioactive substance to enter the brain tissue. A scanning device detects the presence of the radioactive substance and thus can identify an area of tumor, abscess, or hematoma.

GALLIUM SCAN (GAL-le-um skan): Radioactive gallium (gallium citrate) is injected into the bloodstream and is detected in the body using a scanning device that produces an image of the areas where gallium collects. The gallium collects in areas of certain tumors (Hodgkin disease, hepatoma, various adenocarcinomas) and in areas of infection.

POSITRON EMISSION TOMOGRAPHY (POS-i-tron e-MISH-un to-MOG-rah-fe): Radioactive substances (oxygen and glucose are used) that release radioactive particles called positrons are injected into the body and travel to specialized areas such as the brain and heart. Because of the way that the positrons are released, cross-sectional color pictures can be made showing the location of the radioactive substance. This test is used to study disorders of the brain and to diagnose strokes, epilepsy, schizophrenia, and migraine headaches. Also known as a *PET scan*.

PULMONARY PERFUSION SCAN (PUL-mon-ar-e per-FU-shun skan): Radioactive particles are injected intravenously and travel rapidly to areas of the lung that are adequately filled with blood. Regions of obstructed blood flow due to tumor, blood clot, swelling, and inflammation can be seen as nonradioactive areas on the scan.

PULMONARY VENTILATION SCAN (PUL-mon-ar-e ven-ti-LA-shun skan): Radioactive gas (xenon-133) is inhaled, and a special camera detects its presence in the lungs. The scan is used to detect lung segments that fail to fill with the radioactive gas. Lack of filling is usually due to diseases that obstruct the bronchial tubes and air sacs. This scan is also used in the evaluation of lung function prior to surgery.

MYOCARDIAL SCAN (mi-o-KAR-de-al skan): A radioactive substance (thallium chloride-201) is injected intravenously and travels to the heart muscle while the patient is at rest or exercising. A special camera shows up areas that have inadequate collection of radioactive substance, such as areas of blocked blood vessels.

THYROID SCAN (THI-royd skan): A radioactive iodine chemical is injected intravenously and collects in the thyroid gland. A scanning device detects the radioactive substance in the gland, measuring it and producing an image of the gland. The increased or decreased activity of the gland is demonstrated by the gland's capacity to use the radioactive iodine. A thyroid scan is used to evaluate the position, size, and functioning of the thyroid gland.

CLINICAL PROCEDURES

The following procedures are performed on patients to establish a correct diagnosis of an abnormal condition. In some instances, the procedure may also be used to treat the condition.

Pronunciation of each term is given with its meaning. The syllable that gets the accent is in **CAPITAL LETTERS** Terms in SMALL CAPITAL LETTERS are defined elsewhere in the appendix.

ABDOMINOCENTESIS (ab-dom-in-o-sen-TE-sis): See PARACENTESIS.

AMNIOCENTESIS (am-ne-o-sen-TE-sis): Surgical puncture to remove fluid from the sac (amnion) that surrounds the fetus in the uterus. The fluid contains cells from the fetus that can be examined under a microscope.

ASPIRATION (as-peh-RA-shun): The withdrawal of fluid by suction through a needle or tube. The term "aspiration pneumonia" refers to an infection caused by inhalation into the lungs of food or an object.

AUDIOGRAM (AW-de-o-gram): A test using sound waves of various frequencies (e.g., 500 Hz) up to 8000 Hz, which quantifies the extent and type of hearing loss.

AUSCULTATION (aw-skul-TA-shun): The process of listening for sounds produced within the body. This is most often performed with the aid of a stethoscope to determine the condition of the chest or abdominal organs or to detect the fetal heart beat.

BIOPSY (BI-op-se): The removal of a piece of tissue from the body and subsequent examination of the tissue under a microscope. The procedure is performed by means of a surgical knife, needle aspiration, or via endoscopic removal (using a special forceps-like instrument inserted through a hollow flexible tube.) An *excisional biopsy* means that the entire tissue to be examined is removed. An *incisional biopsy* is the removal of only a small amount of tissue, and a *needle biopsy* indicates that tissue is pierced with a hollow needle and fluid is withdrawn for microscopic examination.

BONE MARROW BIOPSY (bon MAH-ro BI-op-se): The removal of a small amount of bone marrow. The cells are then examined under a microscope. Often the hip bone (iliac crest) is used, and the biopsy is helpful in determining the number and type of blood cells in the bone marrow.

BRONCHOSCOPY (brong-KOS-ko-pe): The insertion of a flexible tube (endoscope) into the airway. The lining of the bronchial tubes can be seen, and tissue may be removed for biopsy. The tube is usually inserted through the mouth, but can also be directly inserted into the airway during *mediastinoscopy*. Sedation is required for this procedure.

COLONOSCOPY (ko-lon-OS-ko-pe): The insertion of a flexible tube (endoscope) through the rectum into the colon for visual examination. Biopsy samples may be taken and benign growths, such as polyps, can be removed through the endoscope. The removal of a polyp is called a polypectomy (pol-eh-PEK-to-me).

COLPOSCOPY (kol-POS-ko-pe): The inspection of the cervix through the insertion of a special microscope into the vagina. The vaginal walls are held apart by a speculum so that the cervix (entrance to the uterus) can come into view.

CONIZATION (ko-nih-ZA-shun): The removal of a cone-shaped sample of uterine cervix tissue. This sample is then examined under a microscope for evidence of cancerous growth. The special shape of the tissue sample allows the pathologist to examine the transitional zone of the cervix, where cancers are most likely to develop.

CULDOCENTESIS (kul-do-sen-TE-sis): The insertion of a thin, hollow, needle through the vagina into the cul-de-sac, the space between the rectum and the uterus. Fluid is withdrawn and analyzed for evidence of cancerous cells, infection, or blood cells.

CYSTOSCOPY (sis-TOS-ko-pe): The insertion of a thin tube or cystoscope (endoscope) into the urethra and then into the urinary bladder in order to visualize the bladder. A biopsy of the urinary bladder can be performed through the cystoscope.

DIGITAL RECTAL EXAMINATION (DIG-ih-tal REK-tal eks-am-ih-NA-shun): Physician inserts a gloved finger into the rectum. This procedure is used to detect rectal cancer and as a primary method of detection of prostate cancer.

DILATION AND CURETTAGE (di-LA-shun and kur-ih-TAJ): A series of probes of increasing size are systematically inserted through the vagina into the opening of the cervix. The cervix is thus dilated (widened) so that a curette (spoon-shaped instrument) can be inserted to remove tissue from the lining of the uterus. The tissue is then examined under a microscope. The abbreviation for this procedure is *D and C.*

ELECTROCARDIOGRAPHY (e-lek-tro-kar-de-OG-rah-fe): The connection of electrodes (wires or "leads") to the body to record electric impulses from the heart. The *electrocardiogram* is the actual record produced, and it is useful in discovering abnormalities in heart rhythms and diagnosing heart disorders. Abbreviation is *EKG or ECG.*

ELECTROENCEPHALOGRAPHY (e-lek-tro-en-sef-ah-LOG-rah-fe): The connection electrodes (wires or "leads") to the scalp to record electricity coming from within the brain. The *electroencephalogram* is the actual record produced. It is useful in the diagnosis and monitoring of epilepsy and other brain lesions and in the investigation of neurological disorders. It is also used to evaluate patients in coma (brain inactivity) and in the study of sleep disorders. Abbreviation is *EEG.*

ELECTROMYOGRAPHY (e-lek-tro-mi-OG-rah-fe): The insertion of needle electrodes into muscle to record electrical activity. This procedure detects injuries and diseases that affect muscles and nerves. Abbreviation is *EMG*.

ENDOSCOPY (en-DOS-ko-pe): The insertion of a thin, tube-like instrument (endoscope) into an organ or cavity. The endoscope is placed through a natural opening (the mouth or anus), or into a surgical incision, as through the abdominal wall. Endoscopes contain bundles of glass fibers that carry light (fiberoptic); some instruments are equipped with a small forceps-like device that withdraws a sample of tissue for microscopic study (biopsy). Examples of endoscopy are *bronchoscopy, colonoscopy, esophagoscopy, gastroscopy*, and *laparoscopy*.

ESOPHAGOSCOPY (eh-sof-ah-GOS-ko-pe): The insertion of an endoscope through the mouth and throat into the esophagus. Visual examination of the esophagus to detect ulcers, tumors, or other lesions is thus possible.

ESOPHAGOGASTRODUODENOSCOPY (eh-SOF-ah-go-GAS-tro-du-o-den-NOS-ko-pe): An endoscope is inserted through the mouth into the esophagus, stomach and first part of the small intestine. Also called *EGD*.

EXCISIONAL BIOPSY (ek-SIZ-in-al BI-op-se): See BIOPSY.

FROZEN SECTION (fro-zen SEK-shun): The quick preparation of a biopsy sample for examination during an actual surgical procedure. Tissue is taken from the operating room to the pathology laboratory and frozen. It is then thinly sliced and immediately examined under a microscope to determine if the sample is benign or malignant and to determine the status of margins.

GASTROSCOPY (gas-TROS-ko-pe): The insertion of an endoscope through the esophagus into the stomach for visual examination and/or biopsy of the stomach. When the upper portion of the small intestine is also visualized, the procedure is called *EGD* or *esophagogastroduodenoscopy*.

HOLTER ECG RECORDING (HOL-ter ECG re-KOR-ding): The electrocardiographic record of heart activity over an extended period of time. The Holter monitor is worn by the patient as he/she performs normal daily activities. It detects and aids in management of heart rhythm abnormalities. Also called *Holter monitoring*.

HYSTEROSCOPY (his-ter-OS-ko-pe): The insertion of an endoscope into the uterus for visual examination.

INCISIONAL BIOPSY (in-SIZ-in-al BI-op-se): See BIOPSY.

LAPAROSCOPY (lah-pah-ROS-ko-pe): The insertion of an endoscope into the abdomen. After the patient receives a local anesthetic, a laparoscope is inserted through an incision in the abdominal wall. This procedure affords the doctor a view of the abdominal cavity, the surface of the liver and spleen, and the pelvic region. The laparoscope is often used to perform fallopian tube ligation as a means of preventing pregnancy.

LARYNGOSCOPY (lah-rin-GOS-ko-pe): The insertion of an endoscope into the airway in order to visually examine the voice box (larynx). A laryngoscope transmits a magnified image of the larynx through a system of lenses and mirrors. The procedure can reveal tumors and explain changes in the voice. Sputum samples and tissue biopsies are obtained by using brushes or forceps attached to the laryngoscope.

MEDIASTINOSCOPY (me-de-ah-sti-NOS-ko-pe): The insertion of an endoscope into the mediastinum (the potential space in the chest between the lungs and in front of the heart). A mediastinoscope is inserted through a small incision in the neck while the patient is under anesthesia. This procedure is used to biopsy lymph nodes and to examine other structures within the mediastinum.

NEEDLE BIOPSY (NE-dl BI-op-se): See BIOPSY.

OTOSCOPIC EXAM (o-to-SKOP-ic EK-ZAM): A physician uses an otoscope inserted into the ear canal to check for obstructions (e.g., wax), infection, fluid, and eardrum perforations or scarring.

OPHTHALMOSCOPIC EXAM (of-thal-mo-SKOP-ic ek-ZAM): A physician uses an ophthalmoscope to look directly into the eye, evaluating the lens for cataracts, and the optic nerve, retina, and blood vessels in the back of the eye.

PALPATION (pal-PA-shun): Examination by touch. This is a technique of manual physical examination by which a doctor feels underlying tissues and organs through the skin.

PAP SMEAR (pap smer): The insertion of a cotton swab or wooden spatula into the vagina to obtain a sample of cells from the outer surface of the cervix (neck of the uterus). The cells are then smeared on a glass slide, preserved, and sent to the laboratory for microscopic examination. This test for cervical cancer was developed and named after the late Dr. George Papanicolaou. Results are reported as a Grade I–IV (I = normal, II = inflammatory, III = suspicious of malignancy, IV = malignancy).

PARACENTESIS (pah-rah-sen-TE-sis): Surgical puncture of the membrane surrounding the abdomen (peritoneum) to remove fluid from the abdominal cavity. Fluid is drained for analysis and to prevent its accumulation in the abdomen. Also known as *abdominocentesis*.

PELVIC EXAM (PEL-vik ek-ZAM): Physician examines female sex organs and checks the uterus and ovaries for enlargement, cysts, tumors, or abnormal bleeding. This is also known as an "internal exam."

PERCUSSION (per-KUSH-un): The technique of striking a part of the body with short, sharp taps of the fingers to determine the size, density, and position of the underlying parts by the sound obtained. Percussion is commonly used on the abdomen to examine the liver.

PROCTOSIGMOIDOSCOPY (prok-to-sig-moy-DOS-ko-pe): The insertion of an endoscope through the anus to examine the first 10 to 12 inches of the rectum and colon. When the sigmoid colon is visualized using a longer endoscope, the procedure is called *sigmoidoscopy*. The procedure detects polyps, malignant tumors, and sources of bleeding.

PULMONARY FUNCTION STUDY (PUL-mon-nah-re FUNG-shun STUH-de): The measurement of the air taken into and exhaled from the lungs by means of an instrument called a *spirometer*. The test may be abnormal in patients with asthma, chronic bronchitis, emphysema, and occupational exposures to asbestos, chemicals, and dusts.

SIGMOIDOSCOPY (sig-moy-DOS-ko-pe): See PROCTOSIGMOIDOSCOPY.

STRESS TEST: This is an electrocardiogram taken during exercise. It may reveal hidden heart disease or confirm the cause of cardiac symptoms.

THORACENTESIS (thor-ah-sen-TE-sis): The insertion of a needle into the chest to remove fluid from the space surrounding the lungs (pleural cavity). After injection of a local anesthetic, a hollow needle is placed through the skin and muscles of the back and into the space between the lungs and chest wall. Fluid is then withdrawn by applying suction. Excess fluid (*pleural effusion*) may be a sign of infection or malignancy. This procedure is used for diagnostic studies, to drain a pleural effusion, or to re-expand a collapsed lung (*atelectasis*).

THORACOSCOPY (tho-rah-KOS-ko-pe): The insertion of an endoscope through an incision in the chest in order to visually examine the surface of the lungs.

LABORATORY TESTS

The following laboratory tests are performed on samples of a patient's blood, *plasma* (fluid portion of the blood), *serum* (plasma minus clotting proteins and produced after blood has clotted), urine, feces, *sputum* (mucus coughed up from the lungs), *cerebrospinal fluid* (fluid within the spaces around the spinal cord and brain), and skin.

Pronunciation of each term is given with its meaning. The syllable that gets the accent is in **CAPITAL LETTERS**. Terms in SMALL CAPITAL LETTERS are defined elsewhere in the appendix.

ACID PHOSPHATASE (AH-sid FOS-fah-tas): Measures the amount of an enzyme called *acid phosphatase* in serum. Enzyme levels are elevated in metastatic prostate cancer. Moderate elevations of this enzyme occur in diseases of bone and when breast cancer cells invade bone tissue.

ALBUMIN (al-BU-min): Measures *albumin* (protein) in both serum and in urine. A decrease of albumin in serum indicates disease of the kidneys, malnutrition, or liver disease or may occur in extensive loss of protein in the gut or from the skin, as in a burn. The presence of albumin in the urine (*albuminuria*) indicates malfunction of the kidney.

ALKALINE PHOSPHATASE (AL-kah-lin FOS-fah-tas): Measures the amount of *alkaline phosphatase* (an enzyme found on cell membranes) in serum. Levels are elevated in liver diseases (such as hepatitis and hepatoma), and in bone disease and bone cancer. The laboratory symbol is *alk phos*.

ALPHA-FETOPROTEIN (al-fa-fe-to-PRO-ten): Test for the presence of a protein called alpha-globulin in serum. The protein is normally present in the serum of the fetus, infant, and pregnant women. In fetuses with abnormalities of the brain and spinal cord, the protein leaks into the amniotic fluid surrounding the fetus and is an indicator of spinal tube defect (spina bifida) or anencephaly (lack of brain development). High levels are found in patients with cancer of the liver and other malignancies (testicular and ovarian cancers). Serum levels monitor the effectiveness of cancer treatment. Elevated levels are also seen in benign liver disease such as cirrhosis and viral hepatitis. The laboratory symbol is *AFP*.

ANA: See ANTINUCLEAR ANTIBODY TEST.

ANTINUCLEAR ANTIBODY TEST (an-tih-NU-kle-ar AN-tih-bod-e test): A sample of plasma is tested for the presence of antibodies that are found in patients with systemic lupus erythematosus. Laboratory symbol is *ANA*.

BENCE JONES PROTEIN (BENS jonz PRO-ten): Measures the presence of the Bence Jones protein in serum or urine. Bence Jones protein is a fragment of a normal serum protein, an immunoglobulin, produced by cancerous bone marrow cells (myeloma cells). Normally it is not found in either blood or urine, but in *multiple myeloma* (a malignant condition of bone marrow) high levels of Bence Jones protein are detected in urine and serum.

BILIRUBIN (bil-eh-RU-bin): Measures the amount of *bilirubin*, an orange-brown pigment, in serum and urine. Bilirubin is derived from hemoglobin, the oxygen-carrying protein in red blood cells. Its presence in high concentration in serum and urine causes jaundice (yellow coloration of the skin) and may indicate disease of the liver, obstruction of bile ducts, or a type of anemia that leads to excessive destruction of red blood cells.

BLOOD CHEMISTRY PROFILE: This comprehensive blood test provides information regarding the function of several body systems. Tests include calcium (bones), phosphorus (bones), urea (kidney), creatinine (kidney), bilirubin (liver), SGOT (liver and heart muscle) and SGPT (liver), alkaline phosphatase (liver and bone), globulin (liver and immune disorders), and albumin (liver and kidney). Laboratory symbol is *SMAC*.

BLOOD CULTURE (blud KUL-chur): To test for infection in the bloodstream, a sample of blood is added to a special medium (food) that promotes the growth of microorganisms. The medium is then examined by a medical technologist for evidence of bacteria or other microbes.

BLOOD UREA NITROGEN (blud u-RE-ah NI-tro-jen): Measures the amount of urea (nitrogen-containing waste material) in serum. A high level of serum urea indicates poor kidney function, since it is the kidney's job to remove urea from the bloodstream and filter it into urine. Laboratory symbol is *BUN*.

CALCIUM (KAL-se-um): Measures the amount of calcium in serum, plasma, or whole blood. Low blood levels are associated with abnormal functioning of nerves and muscles, and high blood levels indicate loss of calcium from bones, excessive intake of calcium, disease of the parathyroid glands, or cancer. Laboratory symbol is *Ca*.

CARBON DIOXIDE (KAR-bon di-OK-side): This gas, produced in tissues and eliminated by the lungs, is measured in the blood. Abnormal levels may reflect lung disorders. Laboratory symbol is CO_2.

CARCINOEMBRYONIC ANTIGEN (kar-sih-no-em-bree-ON-ik AN-ti-jen): A plasma test for a protein normally found in the blood of human fetuses and produced in healthy adults only in a very small amount, if at all. High levels of this antigen may be a sign of one of a variety of cancers, especially colon or pancreatic cancer. This test is used to monitor the response of patients to cancer treatment. Laboratory abbreviation is *CEA*.

CEREBROSPINAL FLUID (seh-re-bro-SPI-nal FLU-id): Chemical tests are performed on specimens of cerebrospinal fluid removed by *lumbar puncture*. The fluid is tested for protein, sugar, and blood cells. It is also cultured to detect microorganisms. Abnormal conditions such as meningitis, brain tumor, and encephalitis are detected using this test. Laboratory abbreviation is *CSF*.

CHOLESTEROL (ko-LES-ter-ol): Measures the amount of cholesterol (substance found in animal fats and oils, egg yolks, and milk) in serum or plasma. Normal values vary for age and diet; levels above 200 mg/dl indicate a need for further testing and efforts to reduce cholesterol level, since high levels are associated with hardening of arteries and heart disease. Blood is also tested for the presence of a lipoprotein substance that is a combination of cholesterol and protein. High levels of *HDL* (high-density lipoprotein) cholesterol in the blood are beneficial, since HDL cholesterol promotes the removal and excretion of excess cholesterol from the body, while high levels of low-density lipoprotein (*LDL*) are dangerous.

COMPLETE BLOOD COUNT: Numbers of leukocytes (white blood cells), erythrocytes (red blood cells), and platelets (clotting cells) are determined. The CBC is useful in diagnosing anemia, infection, and blood cell disorders, such as leukemia.

CREATINE KINASE (KRE-ah-tin KI-nas): Serum test to detect levels of creatine kinase, a blood enzyme. Creatine kinase is normally found in heart muscle, brain tissue, and skeletal muscle. The presence of one form (*isoenzyme*) of creatine kinase (either CK-MB or CK2) in the blood is strongly indicative of recent myocardial infarction (heart attack), since the enzyme is released from heart muscle when the muscle is damaged or dying.

CREATININE (kre-AT-tih-nin): Measures the amount of creatinine, a nitrogen-containing waste material, in serum or plasma. It is the most reliable test for kidney function. Since creatinine is normally produced as a protein breakdown product in muscle and excreted by the kidney in urine, an elevation in the creatinine level in the blood indicates a disturbance of kidney function. Elevations are also seen in high protein diets and dehydration.

CREATININE CLEARANCE (kre-AT-ih-nin KLER-ans): Measures the rate at which creatinine is cleared (filtered) by the kidneys from the blood. If creatinine clearance is low, it indicates that the kidneys are not functioning effectively to clear creatinine from the bloodstream and filter it into urine.

CULTURE (KUL-chur): This test identifies microorganisms in a special laboratory medium (fluid, solid, or semisolid material). In *sensitivity* tests, culture plates containing a specific microorganism are prepared, and antibiotic-containing disks are applied to the culture surface. Following overnight incubation, the area surrounding the disk (where growth was inhibited) is measured to determine if the antibiotic is effective against the specific organism.

DIFFERENTIAL (di-fer-EN-shul): See WHITE BLOOD CELL COUNT.

ELECTROLYTES (e-LEK-tro-litz): Tests on serum or whole blood to determine the concentration of *electrolytes* (chemical substances which are capable of conducting an electric current). When dissolved in water, electrolytes break apart into charged particles (*ions*). Positively charged electrolytes are *sodium* (Na^+), *potassium* (K^+), *calcium* (CA^{++}), and *magnesium* (MG^{++}). Negatively charged electrolytes are *chloride* (Cl^-) and *bicarbonate* (HCO_3^-). These charged particles should be present at all times for proper functioning of cells. An electrolyte imbalance occurs when serum concentration is either too high or too low. Calcium balance can affect the bones, kidneys, gastrontestinal tract, and neuromuscular activity, while sodium affects blood pressure, nerve functioning, and fluid levels surrounding cells. Potassium affects heart and muscular activity.

ELECTROPHORESIS: See SERUM PROTEIN ELECTROPHORESIS.

ELISA (eh-LI-zah): A laboratory assay (test) for the presence of antibodies to the AIDS virus. If a patient tests positive, it is likely that his/her blood contains the AIDS virus (HIV or human immunodeficiency virus). The presence of the virus stimulates white blood cells to make antibodies that are detected by the ELISA assay. This is the first test done to detect AIDS infection and is followed by a *Western blot* test to confirm the results. ELISA is an acronym for *enzyme-linked immunosorbent assay*.

ERYTHROCYTE SEDIMENTATION RATE (eh-RITH-ro-sit sed-ih-men-TA-shun rat): Measures the rate at which red blood cells (erythrocytes) in well-mixed venous blood settle to the bottom (sediment) of a test tube. If the rate of sedimentation is markedly slow (elevated sed rate), it may indicate inflammatory conditions, such as rheumatoid arthritis, or conditions that produce excessive proteins in the blood. Laboratory symbols are *ESR* and *sed rate*.

ESTRADIOL (es-tra-DI-ol): A test for the concentration of estradiol, which is a form of estrogen (female hormone) in serum, plasma, or urine.

ESTROGEN RECEPTOR ASSAY (ES-tro-jen re-SEP-to-AS-a): This test, performed at the time of a biopsy, determines if a sample of tumor contains an estrogen receptor protein. The protein, if present on breast cancer cells, combines with estrogen, allowing estrogen to promote the growth of the tumor. Thus, if an estrogen receptor assay test is positive (the protein is present) then treatment with an anti-estrogen drug would retard tumor growth. If the assay is negative (the protein is not present), then the tumor would not be affected by anti-estrogen drug treatment.

GLOBULIN (FLOB-u-lin): Measured in serum, *globulins* are proteins that bind to and destroy foreign substances (antigens). Globulins are made by cells of the immune system. Gamma globulin is one type of globulin that contains antibodies to fight disease.

GLUCOSE (GLU-kos): Measures the amount of glucose (sugar) in serum and plasma. High levels of glucose (*hyperglycemia*) indicate diseases such as diabetes mellitus and hyperthyroidism. Glucose is also measured in urine, and its presence indicates diabetes mellitus.

GLUCOSE TOLERANCE TEST (GLU-kos TOL-er-ans test): In the first part of this test, blood and urine samples are taken after the patient has fasted. Then, a solution of glucose is given by mouth. One-half hour after the glucose is taken, blood and urine samples are obtained again, and are collected every hour for 4 to 5 hours. The test determines how the body uses glucose and can indicate abnormal conditions such as diabetes mellitus, hypoglycemia and liver or adrenal gland dysfunction.

HEMATOCRIT (he-MAT-o-krit): Measures the percentage of red blood cells in the blood. The normal range is 40 to 50 per cent in males and 37 to 47 per cent in females. A low hematocrit indicates anemia. Laboratory symbol is *Hct*.

HEMOGLOBIN ASSAY (HE-mo-glo-bin AS-a): Measures the concentration of hemoglobin in blood. The normal blood hemoglobin ranges are 13.5 to 18.0 gm/dl in adult males and 12.0 to 16.0 gm/dl in adult females. Laboratory symbol is *Hgb*.

HEMOCCULT TEST (he-mo-o-KULT test): A small sample of stool is tested for otherwise inapparent ("occult" means "hidden") traces of blood. The sample is placed on the surface of a collection kit and reacts with a chemical (e.g., guaiac). A positive result may indicate bleeding from polyps, ulcers, or malignant tumors.

HUMAN CHORIONIC GONADOTROPIN (HU-man kor-e-ON-ik go-nad-o-TRO-pin): Measures the concentration of human chorionic gonadotropin (a hormone secreted by cells of the fetal placenta) in urine. It is detected in urine within days after fertilization of egg and sperm cells and provides the basis of the most commonly used pregnancy test. Laboratory symbol is *hCG*.

IMMUNOASSAY (im-u-no-AS-a): A method of testing blood and urine for the concentration of various chemicals, such as hormones, drugs, or proteins. The technique makes use of the immunological reaction between antigens and antibodies. An *assay* is a determination of the amount of any particular substance in a mixture.

PKU TEST: This test determines if the urine of a newborn baby contains substances called *phenylketones*. If so, the condition is called *phenylketonuria* (*PKU*). Phenylketonuria occurs in infants born lacking a specific enyzme. If the enzyme is missing, high levels of *phenylalanine* (an amino acid) accumulate in the blood, affecting the infant's brain and causing mental retardation. This situation is prevented by placing the infant on a special diet that prevents accumulation of phenylalanine in the bloodstream.

PLATELET COUNT (PLAT-let kownt): Determines the number of clotting cells (platelets) in a sample of blood.

POTASSIUM (po-TAHS-e-um): Measures the concentration of potassium in serum. Potassium combines with other minerals (such as calcium) and is an important chemical for proper functioning of muscles, especially the heart muscle. Laboratory symbol is K^+. See also ELECTROLYTES.

PROGESTERONE RECEPTOR ASSAY (pro-JES-ter-on re-SEP-tor AS-a): This test determines if a sample of tumor contains a progesterone receptor protein. If positive, it identifies a tumor that would be responsive to anti-progesterone hormone therapy.

PROSTATE-SPECIFIC ANTIGEN (pros-TAT spe-SI-fic AN-ti-jen): This blood test measures the amount of an antigen that is elevated in all patients with prostatic cancer and in some with an inflamed prostate gland. Laboratory symbol is *PSA*.

PROTEIN ELECTROPHORESIS: See SERUM PROTEIN ELECTROPHORESIS.

PROTHROMBIN TIME (pro-THROM-bin tim): Measures the activity of factors in the blood that participate in clotting. Deficiency of any of these factors can lead to a prolonged prothrombin time and difficulty in blood clotting. The test is important as a monitor for patients who are taking anticoagulants, substances that block the activity of blood clotting factors, and increase the risk of bleeding.

PSA: See PROSTATE-SPECIFIC ANTIGEN.

RED BLOOD CELL COUNT: This test counts the number of erythrocytes in a sample of blood. A low red blood cell count may indicate anemia. A high RBC count can indicate *polycythemia vera*.

RHEUMATOID FACTOR (RU-mah-toyd FAK-tor): Detects an abnormal protein (*rheumatoid factor*) present in the serum of patients with rheumatoid arthritis.

SERUM GLUTAMIC-OXALOACETIC TRANSAMINASE (SE-rum glu-TAM-ik oks-al-ah-SE-tik trans-AM-in-as): Measures the amount of the enzyme *glutamate-oxaloacetate transaminase (aspartate transaminase)* in serum. The enzyme is normally present, but when there is damage to heart (heart attack) or liver cells, it is released by the damaged tissue and accumulates in the blood. Laboratory symbol is *SGOT* or *AST*.

SERUM GLUTAMIC-PYRUVIC TRANSAMINASE (SE-rum glu-TAM-ic pi-RU-vik trans-AM-in-as): Measures the amount of the enzyme *glutamate-pyruvic transaminase (alanine transaminase)* in serum. The enzyme is normally in the blood but accumulates in abnormally high amounts when there is acute damage to liver cells as in hepatitis, infectious mononucleosis, and obstructive jaundice. Laboratory symbol is *SGPT* or *ALT*.

SERUM PROTEIN ELECTROPHORESIS (SE-rum PRO-ten e-lek-tro-for-E-sis): This procedure separates proteins using an electric current. The material tested, such as serum, containing various proteins, is placed on paper or gel or in liquid and, under the influence of an electric current, the proteins separate (-phoresis means separation) so that they can be identified and measured. The procedure is also known as *protein electrophoresis*.

SGOT: See SERUM GLUTAMIC-OXALOACETIC TRANSAMINASE.

SGPT: See SERUM GLUTAMIC-PYRUVIC TRANSAMINASE.

SKIN TESTS: In these tests, substances are applied to the skin or injected under the skin, and the reaction of immune cells in the skin is observed. These tests detect a person's sensitivity to substances such as dust or pollen. They can also indicate if a person has been exposed to the bacteria that cause tuberculosis or diphtheria.

SODIUM: See ELECTROLYTES.

SMAC: See BLOOD CHEMISTRY PROFILE.

SPUTUM TEST (SPU-tum test): Examines mucus that is coughed up from a patient's lungs. The sputum is examined microscopically and chemically, and cultured for the presence of microorganisms.

THYROID FUNCTION TESTS (THI-royd FUNK-shun tests): These tests measure the levels of thyroid hormones, such as *thyroxine* (T_4) and *triiodothyronine* (T_3) in serum. *Thyroid-stimulating hormone (TSH)*, which is produced by the pituitary gland and stimulates the release of T_4 and T_3 from the thyroid gland, can also be measured in serum. These tests aid in the diagnosis of hypo- and hyperthyroidism and are helpful in monitoring response to thyroid treatment.

TRIGLYCERIDES (tri-GLIS-er-idz): Determines the amount of *triglycerides* (fats) in the serum. Elevated triglycerides are considered an important risk factor for the development of heart disease.

URIC ACID (UR-ik AS-id): Measures the amount of *uric acid* (a nitrogen-containing waste material) in the serum and urine. High serum levels indicate a type of arthritis called *gout*. In gout, uric acid accumulates as crystals in joints and in tissues. High levels of uric acid may also cause kidney stones.

URINALYSIS (u-rih-NAL-ih-sis): Examination of urine as an aid in the diagnosis of disease. Routine urinalysis involves observation of unusual color or odor; determining specific gravity (amount of materials dissolved in urine); chemical tests (for protein, sugar, acetone); and microscopic examination for bacteria, blood cells, and sediment. Urinalysis is used to detect abnormal functioning of the kidneys and bladder, infections, abnormal growths, and diabetes mellitus. Laboratory symbol is *UA*.

WESTERN BLOT (WES-tern blot): This test is more specific than the ELISA to detect infection by *HIV* (AIDS virus). A patient's serum is mixed with purified proteins from HIV and the reaction is examined. If the patient has made antibodies to HIV, those antibodies will react with the purified HIV proteins, and the test will be positive.

WHITE BLOOD CELL (WBC) COUNT: Determines the number of leukocytes in the blood. Higher than normal counts can indicate the presence of infection or leukemia. A *differential* is the percentages of different types of white blood cells (neutrophils, eosinophils, basophils, lymphocytes, and monocytes) in a sample of blood. It gives more specific information about leukocytes and aids in diagnosis of allergic diseases, disorders of the immune system, and various forms of leukemia.

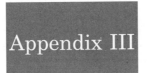

Appendix III

Abbreviations and Symbols

ABBREVIATIONS

abd	Abdomen
AB	Abortion
a.c.	Before meals (*ante cibum*)
ACE	Angiotension converting enzyme (ACE inhibitors are used to treat hypertension)
ACTH	Adrenocorticotropic hormone (secreted by the pituitary gland)
AD	Right ear (*auris dexter*)
ADH	Antidiuretic hormone (secreted by the pituitary gland)
ad lib	Freely as desired (*ad libitum*)
AIDS	Acquired immunodeficiency syndrome
alb	Albumin (protein)
ALL	Acute lymphocytic leukemia
alk phos	Alkaline phosphatase (enzyme elevated in liver disease)
ALS	Amyotrophic lateral sclerosis (Lou Gehrig disease)
ALT	Alanine transaminase (enzyme elevated in liver disease); see SGPT
AML	Acute myelocytic leukemia
AP	Anteroposterior (front to back)
A&P	Auscultation and percussion
aq	Water (*aqua*)
AS	Left ear (*auris sinister*)
ASD	Atrial septal defect
ASHD	Arteriosclerotic heart disease
AST	Aspartate aminotransferase (elevated in liver and heart disease); see SGOT
AU	Both ears (*auris uterque*)
AV	Atrioventricular
A&W	Alive and well
BA	Barium
BaE (BE)	Barium enema
B cells	White blood cells (lymphocytes) produced in the bone marrow
b.i.d.	Twice a day (*bis in die*)
BM	Bowel movement
BP	Blood pressure
BPH	Benign prostatic hyperplasia (hypertrophy)
Broncho	Bronchoscopy
BS	Blood sugar
BSE	Breast self-examination
BUN	Blood urea nitrogen (test of kidney function)
Bx	Biopsy

c̄	With (*cum*)
C1, C2	First, second cervical vertebra
Ca	Calcium; cancer; carcinoma
CABG	Coronary artery bypass graft
CAD	Coronary artery disease
CAPD	Continuous ambulatory peritoneal dialysis
cap	Capsule
CBC	Complete blood count
cc	Cubic centimeter (1/1000 liter)
CCU	Coronary care unit
CF	Cystic fibrosis
Chemo	Chemotherapy
CHF	Congestive heart failure
CIN	Cervical intraepithelial neoplasia
CIS	Carcinoma in situ
cm	Centimeter (1/100 meter)
CML	Chronic myelocytic (myelogenous) leukemia
CNS	Central nervous system
c/o	Complains of
CO₂	Carbon dioxide
COPD	Chronic obstructive pulmonary disease
CP	Cerebral palsy; chest pain
CPD	Cephalopelvic disproportion
CPR	Cardiopulmonary resuscitation
C&S	Culture and sensitivity
CS	Cesarean section
C-section	Cesarean section
CSF	Cerebrospinal fluid
CT	Computed tomography (see CT scan)
CT (CAT) scan	Computed axial tomography (x-ray images in cross-sectional view)
CVA	Cerebrovascular accident (stroke)
CXR	Chest x-ray
D/C	Discontinue; discharge
D&C	Dilation and curettage (of the uterine lining)
DES	Diethylstilbestrol (estrogen causing defects in children whose mothers took the drug during pregnancy)
DJD	Degenerative joint disease
diff	Differential (percentages of types of white blood cells)
DM	Diabetes mellitus
DNA	Deoxyribonucleic acid
DOB	Date of birth
DOE	Dyspnea on exertion
DRE	Digital rectal exam

DT	Delirium tremens (caused by alcohol withdrawal)
DTR	Deep tendon reflex
DVT	Deep vein thrombosis
Dx	Diagnosis
EBV	Epstein-Barr virus (cause of mononucleosis)
ECG (EKG)	Electrocardiogram
ECT	Electroconvulsive therapy
EDC	Estimated date of confinement
EEG	Electroencephalogram
EGD	Esophagogastroduodenoscopy
EMG	Electromyogram
ENT	Ears, nose, throat
Eos	Eosinophil (type of white blood cell)
ER	Emergency room; estrogen receptor
ERCP	Endoscopic retrograde cholangiopancreatography
ESR	Erythrocyte sedimentation rate; see sed. rate
ESRD	End-stage renal disease
ESWL	Extracorporeal shock-wave lithotripsy
ETOH	Ethyl alcohol
FBC	Fasting blood sugar
Fe	Iron
FH	Family history
FHT	Fetal heart tones
FSH	Follicle-stimulating hormone (secreted by the pituitary gland)
F/u	Follow-up
5-FU	5-Fluorouracil (drug used in cancer chemotherapy)
FUO	Fever of unknown origin
Fx	Fracture
g (gm)	Gram
Ga	Gallium (element used in nuclear medicine diagnostic tests)
GB	Gallbladder
GERD	Gastroesophageal reflux disease
GH	Growth hormone (secreted by the pituitary gland)
GI	Gastrointestinal
Grav. 1,2	First, second pregnancy
gt, gtt	Drop, drops
GTT	Glucose tolerance test
GU	Genitourinary
GYN	Gynecology

H	Hydrogen
h	Hour
HBV	Hepatitis B virus
HCG	Human chorionic gonadotropin (secreted during pregnancy)
HCT (hct)	Hematocrit
HEENT	Head, ears, eyes, nose, and throat
HD	Hemodialysis (artificial kidney machine)
HDL	High-density lipoproteins (associated with decreased incidence of coronary artery disease)
Hg	Mercury
HGB (hgb)	Hemoglobin
HIV	Human immunodeficiency virus
h/o	History of
H_2O	Water
HPV	Human papilloma virus
HRT	Hormone replacement therapy
h.s.	At bedtime (*hora somni*)
HSG	Hysterosalpingogram
HSV-1,2	Herpes simplex virus type 1, 2
HTN	Hypertension (high blood pressure)
Hx	History
I	Iodine
I&D	Incision and drainage
ICU	Intensive care unit
IDDM	Insulin-dependent diabetes mellitus (type I)
IM	Intramuscular
INH	Isoniazid (drug to treat tuberculosis)
I&O	Intake and output (measurement of patient's fluids)
IOL	Intraocular lens (implant)
IUD	Intrauterine device
IV	Intravenous
IVP	Intravenous pyelogram
K^+	Potassium
kg	Kilogram (1000 grams)
KUB	Kidneys, ureters, bladder (x-ray test)
L	Liter; lower
L	Left
L1, L2	First, second lumbar vertebra
LA	Left atrium
lat	Lateral
LB	Large bowel

LD, LDH	Lactate dehydrogenase (elevations associated with heart attacks)
LDL	Low-density lipoproteins (high levels associated with heart disease)
LE	Lupus erythematosus
LEEP	Loop electrosurgical excising procedure
LES	Lower esophageal sphincter
LLQ	Left lower quadrant (of the abdomen)
LMP	Last menstrual period
LP	Lumbar puncture
LTB	Laryngotracheal bronchitis
LUQ	Left upper quadrant (of the abdomen)
LV	Left ventricle
LVH	Left ventricular hypertrophy
L&W	Living and well
lymphs	Lymphocytes
lytes	Electrolytes
m	Meter
MCH	Mean corpuscular hemoglobin (amount in each red blood cell)
MCHC	Mean corpuscular hemoglobin concentration (amount per unit of blood)
MCV	Mean corpuscular volume (size of individual red blood cell)
MD	Medical doctor; muscular dystrophy
mets	Metastases
mg	Milligram (1/1000 gram)
Mg	Magnesium
MH	Marital history; mental health
MI	Myocardial infarction (heart attack)
ml	Milliliter (1/1000 liter)
mm	Millimeter (1/1000 meter)
mm Hg	Millimeters of mercury (measurement of blood pressure)
mono	Monocytes (type of white blood cell)
MRA	Magnetic resonance angiography
MRI	Magnetic resonance imaging
MS	Mitral stenosis; multiple sclerosis; musculoskeletal
MVP	Mitral valve prolapse
Na$^+$	Sodium
NB	Newborn
NED	No evidence of disease
NG tube	Nasogastric tube
NIDDM	Non-insulin dependent diabetes mellitus (type II diabetes)
NKDA	No known drug allergies

NPO	Nothing by mouth (*nulli per os*)
NSAID	Non-steroidal anti-inflammatory drug
NSR	Normal sinus rhythm (of the heart)
NTP	Normal temperature and pressure
O₂	Oxygen
OA	Osteoarthritis
OB	Obstetrics
OD	Right eye (*oculus dexter*); doctor of optometry
OPD	Outpatient department
OR	Operating room
ORIF	Open reduction, internal fixation (to set a broken bone)
OS	Left eye (*oculus sinister*)
os	Mouth
OU	Both eyes (*oculus uterque*)
p̄	After
P	Plan; posterior; pulse; phosphorus
PA	Posteroanterior (back to front)
PAC	Premature atrial contraction
PaCO₂	Arterial pressure of carbon dioxide in the blood; also written PCO_2
palp	Palpable; palpation (examine by touch)
PaO₂	Arterial pressure of oxygen in the blood; also written PO_2
PAP smear	Papanicolaou smear (microscopic examination of cells from the cervix and vagina)
Para 1,2	Woman having produced one, two viable offspring; unipara, bipara
p.c.	After meals (*post cibum*)
PD	Peritoneal dialysis
PDN	Private duty nurse
PE	Physical examination
per	by
PERRLA	Pupils equal, round, and reactive to light and accommodation
PET	Positron emission tomography
PE tube	Ventilating tube for the eardrum
PFT	Pulmonary function test
pH	Hydrogen ion concentration (measurement of acidity or alkalinity of a solution)
PH	Past history
PI	Present illness
PID	Pelvic inflammatory disease
PKU	Phenylketonuria (test for lack of an enzyme in infants)
p.m.	Afternoon (*post meridian*)

PMH	Past medical history
PND	Paroxysmal nocturnal dyspnea
PNS	Peripheral nervous system
p/o	Postoperative
p.o.	By mouth (*per os*)
polys	Polymorphonuclear leukocytes (neutrophils)
poplit	Popliteal (behind the knee)
post-op	After operation
p.p.	After meals (*post prandial*); after birth (*post partum*)
PPBS	Postprandial blood sugar
PPD	Purified protein derivative (skin test for tuberculosis)
PR	Per rectum
pre-op	Before operation
prep	Prepare for
p.r.n.	As needed (*pro re nata*)
procto	Proctoscopy (visual examination of the anus and rectum)
Pro. time	Prothrombin time (test of blood clotting)
PSA	Prostate-specific antigen
PT	Physical therapy; prothrombin time
pt	Patient
PTA	Prior to admission (to hospital)
PTCA	Percutaneous transluminal coronary angioplasty (balloon angioplasty)
PTH	Parathyroid hormone
PTR	Patient to return
PTT	Partial thromboplastin time (test of blood clotting)
PVC	Premature ventricular contraction (abnormal heart rhythm)
q	Every (*quaque*)
q.d.	Each day (*quaque die*)
q.h.	Each hour (*quaque hora*)
q2h	Each two hours (*quaque secunda hora*)
q.i.d.	Four times a day (*quater in die*)
q.n.	Each night (*quaque nox*)
q.n.s.	Quantity not sufficient (*quantum non satis*)
q.s.	Quantity sufficient (*quantum satis*)
qt	Quart
R, r, rt	Right; respiration
R	Right
RA	Rheumatoid arthritis
RBC, rbc	Red blood cell
RIA	Radioimmunoassay (minute quantities are measured)
RLQ	Right lower quadrant (of the abdomen)
R/O	Rule out

ROM	Range of motion
ROS	Review of systems
RP	Retrograde pyelogram (urogram)
RR	Recovery room; respiration rate
RRR	Regular rate and rhythm (of the heart)
RT	Radiation therapy
RUQ	Right upper quadrant (of the abdomen)
RV	Right ventricle (of the heart)
Rx	Treatment (recipe)
s̄	Without (*sine*)
S1, S2	First, second sacral vertebra
S-A node	Sinoatrial node (pacemaker of the heart)
SBFT	Small bowel follow-through (x-rays of the small intestine with contrast)
sed. rate	Erythrocyte sedimentation rate (time it takes red blood cells to settle out of blood)
segs	Segmented white blood cells (granulocytes)
s.gl.	Without glasses
SGOT (AST)	Serum glutamic-oxaloacetic transaminase (high blood levels associated with liver and heart disease)
SGPT (ALT)	Serum glutamic-pyruvic transaminase (high blood levels associated with liver disease)
SH	Social history
sig	Let it be labeled
SLE	Systemic lupus erythematosus
SOAP	Subjective (symptoms perceived by the patient) data, Objective (exam findings) data, Assessment (evaluation of condition), Plan (goals for treatment)
SOB	Shortness of breath
S/P	Status post (previous disease condition)
SPECT	Single photon emission computed tomography
SpGr	Specific gravity
sq	Subcutaneous
Staph	Staphylococci (bacteria)
stat	Immediately (*statim*)
STD	Sexually transmitted disease
Strep	Streptococci (bacteria)
Sx	Symptoms
T	Temperature
T1, T2	First, second thoracic vertebra
T$_3$	Triiodothyronine (thyroid gland hormone)
T$_4$	Thyroxine (thyroid gland hormone)
T&A	Tonsillectomy and adenoidectomy

TAB	Therapeutic abortion
tab	Tablet
TAH	Total abdominal hysterectomy
TB	Tuberculosis
T cells	Lymphocytes originating in the thymus gland
TEE	Transesophageal echocardiogram
TIA	Transient ischemic attack
t.i.d.	Three times a day
TLC	Total lung capacity
TM	Tympanic membrane
TNM	Tumor, nodes, metastasis (staging system for cancer)
tomos	Tomograms (x-ray images to show an organ in depth)
TPN	Total parenteral nutrition
TPR	Temperature, pulse, respiration
TSH	Thyroid-stimulating hormone (secreted by the pituitary gland)
TUR, TURP	Transurethral resection of the prostate gland
TVH	Total vaginal hysterectomy
Tx	Treatment
UA, U/A	Urinalysis
UE	Upper extremity
UGI	Upper gastrointestinal
umb	Navel (umbilical cord region)
ung	Ointment
U/O	Urine output
URI	Upper respiratory infection
u/s	Ultrasound
UTI	Urinary tract infection
UV	Ultraviolet
VA	Visual acuity
VC	Vital capacity (of lungs)
VCUG	Voiding cystourethrogram
VF	Visual field
v/s	Vital signs
VSD	Ventricular septal defect
V tach, V.T.	Ventricular tachycardia (abnormal heart rhythm)
WBC, wbc	White blood cell; white blood count
WDWN	Well developed, well nourished
W/C	Wheelchair
wd	Wound
WNL	Within normal limits

WT, wt	Weight
w/u	Work-up
y/o, yrs	Year(s) old

SYMBOLS

=	Equal
≠	Unequal
+	Positive
−	Negative
↑	Above, increase
↓	Below, decrease
♀	Female
♂	Male
→	To (in direction of)
>	Is greater than
<	Is less than
1°, 2°	Primary, secondary to
ʒ	Dram
℥	Ounce

Glossary of Medical Terms

Pronunciation of each term is given with its meaning.* The syllable that gets the accent is in CAPITAL LETTERS. Terms in SMALL CAPITAL LETTERS are defined elsewhere in the glossary.

ABDOMEN (AB-do-men): space below the chest, containing organs such as the stomach, liver, intestines, and gallbladder. Also called the abdominal cavity, the abdomen lies between the diaphragm and the pelvis (hip bone).

ABDOMINAL (ab-DOM-i-nal): pertaining to the abdomen.

ABDOMINAL CAVITY (ab-DOM-i-nal KAV-i-te): see ABDOMEN.

ABNORMAL (ab-NOR-mal): pertaining to being away (AB-) from the norm; irregular.

ACQUIRED IMMUNODEFICIENCY SYNDROME (ah-KWI-erd im-u-no-deh-FISH-en-se SIN-drom): suppression or deficiency of the immune response caused by exposure to the human immunodeficiency virus (HIV).

ACROMEGALY (ak-ro-MEG-ah-le): enlargement of extremities as a result of thickening of bones and soft tissues; caused by excessive secretion of growth hormone from the pituitary gland (after completion of puberty).

ACUTE (ah-KUT): sharp, sudden, intense for a short period of time.

ADENITIS (ad-en-NI-tis): inflammation of a gland.

ADENOCARCINOMA (ah-deh-no-kar-sih-NO-mah): cancerous tumor derived from glandular cells.

ADENOIDS (AD-eh-noidz): enlarged lymphatic tissue in the upper part of the throat near the nasal passageways.

ADENOIDECTOMY (ah-deh-noyd-EK-to-me): removal of ADENOIDS.

ADENOMA (ah-deh-NO-mah): benign tumor of glandular cells.

ADENOPATHY (ah-deh-NOP-ah-the): disease of glands. Often this term means enlargement of lymph nodes (which are not true glands, but collections of lymphatic tissue).

ADNEXA UTERI (ad-NEKS-ah U-ter-i): accessory structures of the uterus (ovaries, and fallopian tubes).

ADRENAL CORTEX (ad-DRE-nal KOR-teks): outermost part of the adrenal gland. The adrenal cortex secretes steroid hormones such as glucocorticoids (cortisone).

ADRENAL GLANDS (ah-DRE-nal glanz): two endocrine glands, each above a kidney. The adrenal glands produce hormones such as adrenalin (epinephrine) and hydrocortisone (cortisol).

ADRENALECTOMY (ah-dre-nal-EK-to-me): removal (excision) of adrenal glands.

ADRENOPATHY (ah-dre-NOP-a-the): disease of adrenal glands.

AIDS: see ACQUIRED IMMUNODEFICIENCY SYNDROME.

AIR SACS (ayr-saks): thin-walled sacs within the lung. Inhaled oxygen passes into the blood from the sacs, and carbon dioxide passes out from the blood into the sacs to be exhaled.

---

*No diacritical (accent) marks are used except ī to indicate the long i in words ending in -CYTE.

ALBUMINURIA (al-bu-men-U-re-ah): albumin (protein) in the urine; indicating malfunction of the kidney.

ALLERGIST (AL-er-jist): medical doctor specializing in identifying and treating abnormal sensitivity to foreign substances such as pollen, dust, foods, and drugs.

ALOPECIA (ah-lo-PE-shah): loss of hair; baldness.

ALVEOLAR (al-VE-o-lar): pertaining to air sacs (alveoli) within the lungs.

ALVEOLUS (al-ve-O-lus): an air sac within the lung (pl. alveoli).

ALZHEIMER DISEASE (ALTZ-hi-mer di-ZEZ): deterioration of mental capacity (irreversible dementia) marked by intellectual deterioration, disorganization of personality, and difficulties in carrying out tasks of daily living.

AMENORRHEA (a-men-o-RE-ah): absence of menstrual periods.

AMNIOCENTESIS (am-ne-o-sen-TE-sis): surgical puncture to remove fluid from the amnion (sac surrounding the developing fetus).

ANAL (A-nal): pertaining to the anus (opening of the rectum to the outside of the body).

ANALYSIS (ah-NAL-ih-sis): separating a substance into its component parts.

ANEMIA (ah-NE-me-ah): reduced amount of oxygen to body tissues. This may result from deficiencies and abnormalities of red blood cells or loss of blood. Literally, anemia means lacking (AN-) in blood (-EMIA).

ANEMIC (ah-NE-mik): pertaining to ANEMIA.

ANESTHESIOLOGIST (an-es-the-ze-OL-o-jist): medical doctor specializing in administering agents capable of bringing about loss of sensation and consciousness.

ANESTHESIOLOGY (an-es-the-ze OL-o-je): study of how to administer agents capable of bringing about loss of sensation and consciousness.

ANEURYSM (AN-u-rizm): localized widening of the wall of an artery, vein, or of the heart. From ANA- meaning "throughout" and EURUS meaning "wide."

ANGINA (an-JI-nah): sharp pain in the chest resulting from a decrease in blood supply to heart muscle; also called angina pectoris (chest).

ANGIOGRAPHY (an-je-OG-rah-fe): x-ray recording of blood vessels after contrast is injected.

ANGIOPLASTY (AN-je-o-plas-te): surgical repair of a blood vessel. A tube (catheter) is placed in a clogged artery and a balloon in the end of the tube is inflated to flatten the clogged material against the wall of the artery. This enlarges the opening of the artery so that more blood can pass through. Also called balloon angioplasty.

ANKYLOSING SPONDYLITIS (ang-ki-LO-sing spon-dih-LI-tis): chronic inflammation of the vertebrae (backbones) with stiffening of spinal joints so that movement becomes increasingly painful.

ANKYLOSIS (ang-ki-LO-sis): stiffening and immobility of a joint due to injury, disease, or surgical procedure.

ANOMALY (an-NOM-ah-le): an irregularity; deviation from the normal. A congenital anomaly (irregularity) is present at birth.

ANTE MORTEM (AN-te MOR-tem): before death.

ANTE NATAL (AN-te NA-tal): before birth.

ANTE PARTUM (AN-te PAR-tum): before birth.

ANTERIOR (an-TE-re-or): located in the front (of the body or of a structure).

ANTIARRHYTHMIC (an-te-ah-RITH-mik): pertaining to a drug that works against or prevents abnormal heartbeats (arrhythmias).

ANTIBIOTIC (an-tih-bi-OT-ik): pertaining to against germ or bacterial life.

ANTIBODY (AN-tih-bod-e): a substance that works against (ANTI-) germs ("bodies" of infection). Antibodies are produced by white blood cells when germs (antigens) enter the bloodstream.

ANTICOAGULANT (an-tih-ko-AG-u-lant): drug that prevents clotting (coagulation). Anticoagulants are given when there is danger of clots forming in blood vessels.

ANTIGEN (AN-tih-jen): foreign agent (germ) that stimulates white blood cells to make antibodies. Antigens are then destroyed by the antibodies.

ANTIHYPERTENSIVE (an-ti-hi-per-TEN-siv): drug that reduces high blood pressure.

ANURIA (an-U-re-ah): no urine formation by the kidney.

ANUS (A-nus): opening of the rectum to the surface of the body; solid wastes (feces) leave the body through the anus.

AORTA (a-OR-tah): largest artery; it leads from the lower left chamber of the heart to arteries all over the body.

AORTIC STENOSIS (a-OR-tik steh-NO-sis): narrowing of the aorta.

APEX (A-peks): pointed end of an organ. Plural is apices (A-pih-sez).

APHAKIA (ah-FA-ke-ah): absence of the lens of the eye.

APNEA (AP-ne-ah): not (A-) able to breathe (PNEA).

APPENDECTOMY (ap-en-DEK-to-me): removal of the appendix.

APPENDICITIS (ap-en-dih-SI-tis): inflammation of the appendix.

APPENDIX (ah-PEN-dikz): small sac that hangs from the juncture of the small and large intestines in the right lower quadrant of the abdomen. Its function is unknown.

AREOLA (ah-RE-o-lah): dark, pigmented area around the nipple of the breast.

ARRHYTHMIA (a-RITH-me-ah): abnormal heart rhythm.

ARTERIOLE (ar-TER-e-ol): a small artery.

ARTERIOSCLEROSIS (ar-ter-e-o-skle-RO-sis): hardening of arteries. The most common form is *atherosclerosis,* which is hardening of arteries caused by collection of fatty, cholesterol-like deposits (plaque) in arteries.

ARTERY (AR-ter-e): largest blood vessel. Arteries carry blood away from the heart.

ARTHRALGIA (ar-THRAL-je-ah): pain in a joint.

ARTHRITIS (ar-THRI-tis): inflammation of a joint.

ARTHROCENTESIS (ar-thro-sen-TE-sis): surgical puncture to remove fluid from a joint.

ARTHROGRAM (AR-thro-gram): x-ray record of a joint.

ARTHROPATHY (ar-THROP-ah-the): disease of joints.

ARTHROSCOPE (AR-thro-skop): an instrument to examine the inside of a joint.

ARTHROSCOPY (ar-THROS-ko-pe): process of visual examination of a joint.

ARTHROSIS (ar-THRO-sis): abnormal condition of a joint.

ASCITES (ah-SI-tez): abnormal collection of fluid in the abdomen.

ASPHYXIA (as-FIK-se-ah): deficiency of oxygen in the blood and increase in carbon dioxide in blood and tissues. Major symptom is a complete absence of breathing.

ASTHMA (AZ-mah): difficult breathing caused by spasm of bronchial tubes or swelling of their mucous membrane lining.

ATELECTASIS (ah-teh-LEK-tah-sis): collapsed lung (ATEL meaning "incomplete"; -ECTASIS meaning "widening or dilation").

ATHEROSCLEROSIS (ah-theh-ro-skle-RO-sis): see ARTERIOSCLEROSIS.

ATRIUM (A-tre-um): upper chamber of the heart (pl. atria).

ATROPHY (AT-ro-fe): decrease in size of an organ.

AUDITORY CANAL (AW-dih-to-re kah-NAL): passageway leading into the ear from the outside of the body.

AUDITORY NERVE (AW-dih-to-re nurve): carries messages from the inner ear to the brain, making hearing possible.

AURA (AW-rah): a strange sensation coming before more definite symptoms of illness. Often precedes a migraine headache, warning the patient that an attack is beginning.

AURAL DISCHARGE (AW-rah DIS-charge): fluid or material from the ear.

AUTOPSY (AW-top-se): examination of a dead body to discover the actual cause of death. Also called a post mortem exam or necropsy. Literally, to see (-OPSY) with one's own (AUTO-) eyes.

AXIAL (AKS-e-al): pertaining to an axis (a line through the center of a body or about which a structure revolves).

AXILLARY (AKS-ih-lar-e): pertaining to the armpit or underarm.

BACTERIUM (bak-TE-re-um): a type of one-celled organism, whose genetic material (DNA) is not organized within a nucleus (pl. bacteria).

BALANITIS (bah-lah-NI-tis): inflammation of the penis.

BARIUM (BAH-re-um): substance used as an opaque (x-rays can't pass through it) contrast medium for x-ray examination of the digestive tract.

BARIUM ENEMA (BAH-re-um EN-eh-mah): x-ray image of the lower digestive tract after injecting a solution of barium into the rectum.

BARIUM MEAL (SWALLOW) (BAH-re-um mel): x-ray image of the upper digestive tract after swallowing a solution of barium.

BENIGN (be-NIN): not cancerous; a tumor that does not spread and is limited in growth.

BENIGN PROSTATIC HYPERPLASIA (be-NIN pro-STAH-tik hi-per-PLA-ze-ah): non-malignant enlargement of the prostate gland.

BILATERAL (bi-LAT-er-al): pertaining to two (both) sides.

BILE (bīl): a yellow or orange fluid produced by the liver. It breaks up large fat globules and helps the digestion of fats.

BILE DUCT (bīl dukt): tube that carries bile from the liver and gallbladder to the intestine.

BILIRUBIN (bil-ih-RU-bin): a red blood cell pigment excreted with bile from the liver into the intestine.

BIOLOGY (bi-OL-o-je): study of life.

BIOPSY (BI-op-se): process of viewing living tissue under a microscope.

BLADDER (BLAD-der): see URINARY BLADDER.

BONE (bōn): hard, rigid type of connective tissue that makes up most of the skeleton. It is composed of calcium salts.

BONE MARROW (bōn MAH-ro): soft, sponge-like material in the inner part of bones. Blood cells are made in the bone marrow.

BRADYCARDIA (bra-de-KAR-de-ah): slow heartbeat.

BRAIN (brān): organ in the head that controls the activities of the body.

BREAST (brest): one of two glandular organs in front of the chest. The breasts produce milk after childbirth.

BRONCHIAL TUBE (BRONG-ke-al tube): one of two tubes that carry air from the windpipe to the lungs. Also called a bronchus (pl. bronchi).

BRONCHIOLE (BRONG-ke-OL): small bronchial tube.

BRONCHIOLITIS (brong-ke-o-LI-tis): inflammation of bronchioles.

BRONCHITIS (brong-KI-tis): inflammation of bronchial tubes.

BRONCHOSCOPE (BRONG-ko-skop): instrument to visually examine bronchial tubes.

BRONCHOSCOPY (bron-KOS-ko-pe): visual examination of bronchial tubes by passing an endoscope through the trachea (windpipe) into the bronchi.

BRONCHUS (BRONG-kus): see BRONCHIAL TUBE.

BURSA (BUR-sah): sac of fluid near a joint; pl. bursae (BUR-see).

CALCANEUS (kal-KA-ne-us): heel bone.

CALCULUS (KAL-ku-lus): a stone; pl. calculi (KAL-ku-li).

CAPILLARY (KAP-il-lar-e): smallest blood vessel (pl. capillaries).

CARBON DIOXIDE (KAHR-bon di-OK-sid): an odorless, colorless gas formed in tissues and eliminated by the lungs.

CARCINOMA (kar-sih-NO-mah): cancerous tumor. Carcinomas form from epithelial cells, which line the internal organs as well as cover the outside of the body.

CARDIAC (KAR-de-ak): pertaining to the heart.

CARDIOLOGIST (kar-de-OL-o-jist): physician specializing in the study of the heart and heart disease.

CARDIOLOGY (kar-de-OL-o-je): study of the heart.

CARDIOMEGALY (kar-de-o-MEG-ah-le): enlargement of the heart.

CARDIOMYOPATHY (kar-de-o-mi-OP-ah-the): disease of heart muscle.

CARDIOVASCULAR SURGEON (kar-de-o-VAS-ku-lar SUR-jin): specialist in operating on the heart and blood vessels.

CARPALS (KAR-palz): wrist bones.

CARPAL TUNNEL SYNDROME (KAR-pal TUN-el SIN-drom): a group of symptoms resulting from compression of the median nerve in the wrist. Symptoms include tingling, pain, and burning sensations in the hand and wrist.

CARTILAGE (KAR-tih-lij): flexible, fibrous connective tissue, found attached to bones and at the ends of bones at the joints.

CATARACT (KAT-ah-raht): clouding of the lens of the eye.

CAT SCAN (kat scan): computerized axial tomography. See CT SCAN.

CELL (sel): smallest unit or part of an organ.

CELLULITIS (sel-u-LI-tis): inflammation of soft tissue under the skin; marked by swelling, redness, and pain and caused by bacterial infection.

CEPHALGIA (seh-FAL-je-ah): headache. Shortened form of cephalalgia.

CEPHALIC (seh-FAL-ik): pertaining to the head.

CEREBELLAR (ser-eh-BEL-ar): pertaining to the cerebellum.

CEREBELLUM (ser-eh-BEL-um): lower, back part of the brain that coordinates muscle movement and balance.

CEREBRAL (se-RE-bral or SER-e-bral): pertaining to the CEREBRUM.

CEREBROVASCULAR ACCIDENT (seh-re-bro-VAS-ku-lar AK-sih-dent): a disorder of blood vessels within the cerebrum. It results from inadequate blood supply to the brain. See also STROKE.

CEREBRUM (seh-RE-brum): largest part of the brain. It controls thought processes, hearing, speech, vision, and body movements.

CERVICAL (SER-vi-kal): pertaining to the neck of the body or the neck (cervix) of the uterus.

CERVICAL REGION (SER-vi-kal RE-jin): seven backbones in area of the neck.

CERVICAL VERTEBRA (SER-vi-kal VER-teh-brah): a backbone in the neck.

CERVIX (SER-viks): the lower, neck-like portion of the uterus opening into the vagina.

CESAREAN SECTION (seh-ZAR-re-an SEK-shun): incision of the uterus to remove the fetus at birth.

CHEMOTHERAPY (ke-mo-THER-ah-pe): treatment with drugs; most often used in treatment for cancer.

CHOLECYSTECTOMY (ko-le-sis-TEK-to-me): removal of the gallbladder.

CHOLEDOCHOTOMY (ko-led-o-KOT-o-me): incision of the common bile duct.

CHOLELITHIASIS (ko-le-lih-THI-ah-sis): abnormal condition of gallstones.

CHONDROMA (kon-DRO-mah): benign tumor of cartilage.

CHRONIC (KRON-ik): lasting over a long period of time.

CHRONIC OBSTRUCTIVE PULMONARY DISEASE (KRON-ik ob-STRUK-tiv PUL-mo-na-re DEH-zes): chronic limitation in airflow into and out of the body; includes chronic bronchitis, ASTHMA, and EMPHYSEMA.

CIRCULATORY SYSTEM (SER-ku-lah-tor-e SIS-tem): organs (heart and blood vessels) that carry blood throughout the body.

CIRRHOSIS (seh-RO-sis): liver disease with deterioration of liver cells; often caused by alcoholism and poor nutrition.

CLAVICLE (KLAV-ih-kuhl): collar bone.

CLINICAL (KLIN-eh-kal): pertaining to the bedside or clinic; involving patient care.

COCCYGEAL (kok-sih-JE-al): pertaining to the tailbone (coccyx).

COCCYGEAL REGION (kok-sih-JE-al RE-jin): four fused (joined together) bones at the base of the spinal column (backbone).

COCCYX (KOK-siks): tailbone.

COLITIS (ko-LI-tis): inflammation of the colon (large intestine).

COLON (KO-lon): large intestine (bowel).

COLONIC POLYPOSIS (ko-LON-ik pol-ih-PO-sis): growths or masses protruding from the mucous membrane lining the colon.

COLONOSCOPY (ko-lon-OS-ko-pe): visual examination of the colon.

COLORECTAL SURGEON (ko-lo-REK-tal SUR-jin): physician specializing in operating on the colon and rectum.

COLOSTOMY (ko-LOS-to-me): opening of the colon to the outside of the body.

COLPOSCOPY (kol-POS-ko-pe): visual examination of the vagina and cervix.

CONCUSSION (kon-KUS-un): loss of consciousness resulting from a blow to the head.

CONGENITAL ANOMALY (con-JEN-ih-tal ah-NOM-ah-le): see ANOMALY.

CONGESTIVE HEART FAILURE (kon-JES-tiv hart FAIL-ur): the heart is unable to pump its required amount of blood resulting in inadequate oxygen to body cells.

CONIZATION (ko-nih-ZA-shun): removal of a wedge-shaped piece (cone) of tissue from the cervix as diagnosis and treatment of early cancer of the cervix.

CONJUNCTIVA (kon-junk-TI-vah): thin protective membrane over the front of the eye and attached to the eyelids.

CONJUNCTIVITIS (kon-junk-ti-VI-tis): inflammation of the CONJUNCTIVA.

CONNECTIVE TISSUE (kon-NEK-tiv TIS-u): fibrous tissue that supports and connects internal organs, bones, and walls of blood vessels.

CORIUM (KOR-e-um): middle layer of the skin below the epidermis; DERMIS.

CORNEA (KOR-ne-ah): transparent layer over the front of the eye. It bends light to focus it on sensitive cells (retina) at the back of the eye.

CORONAL PLANE (kor-O-nal playn): see FRONTAL PLANE.

CORONARY (KOR-on-ary): pertaining to the heart. Coronary arteries branch from the aorta (largest artery) to bring oxygen-rich blood to the heart muscle.

CORTEX (KOR-teks): outer part of an organ; pl. cortices (KOR-teh-sez).

CORTISOL (KOR-tih-sol): anti-inflammatory hormone secreted by the adrenal cortex.

COSTOCHONDRITIS (kos-to-kon-DRI-tis): inflammation of a rib and its cartilage.

COSTOCHONDRAL (kos-to-KON-dral): pertaining to a rib and its cartilage.

CRANIAL CAVITY (KRA-ne-al KAV-ih-te): the space surrounded by the skull and containing the brain and other organs.

CRANIOTOMY (kra-ne-OT-o-me): incision of the skull.

CRANIUM (KRA-ne-um): skull.

CREATININE (kre-AT-tih-nin): nitrogen-containing waste that is removed from the blood by the kidney and excreted in urine.

CROHN DISEASE (kron dih-zes): inflammation of the gastrointestinal tract (often the ILEUM); marked by bouts of diarrhea, abdominal cramping, and fever. Along with ulcerative colitis, it is a type of INFLAMMATORY BOWEL DISEASE.

CRYPTORCHISM (kript-OR-kism): undescended (CRYPT- means "hidden") testicle. The testicle is not in the scrotal sac at birth.

CT SCAN: computed tomography. A series of x-ray images that show organs in cross-section (transverse view). Also called a CAT SCAN.

CUSHING SYNDROME (KOOSH-ing SIN-drom): symptoms produced by an excess of cortisol from the adrenal cortex; marked by moon face, fatty swellings, and weakness.

CYSTITIS (sis-TI-tis): inflammation of the urinary bladder.

CYSTOSCOPE (SIS-to-skop): instrument (endoscope) to view the urinary bladder.

CYSTOSCOPY (sis-TOS-ko-pe): visual examination of the urinary bladder.

CYTOLOGY (si-TOL-o-je): study of cells.

DÉBRIDEMENT (de-BREED-ment): removal of diseased tissue from the skin.

DEMENTIA (deh-MEN-shah): loss of memory and mental abilities.

DERMATITIS (der-mah-TI-tis): inflammation of the skin.

DERMATOLOGIST (der-mah-TOL-o-jist): physician specializing in the skin and its diseases.

DERMATOSIS (der-mah-TO-sis): any abnormal condition of the skin.

DERMIS (DER-mis): fibrous middle layer of the skin below the epidermis. It contains nerves and blood vessels, hair roots, oil and sweat glands; CORIUM.

DIABETES MELLITUS (di-ah-BE-tez MEL-li-tus): disorder marked by deficient INSULIN in the blood. This causes sugar to remain in the blood rather than entering cells. Named from a Greek word meaning "siphon," through which water passes easily, one symptom of diabetes is frequent urination (polyuria). *Type I* or *insulin-dependent diabetes mellitus* often affects younger people and means that patients require injections of insulin. *Type II* or *non-insulin dependent diabetes mellitus* means that insulin is not adequately or appropriately secreted. Type II diabetes has a tendency to develop later in life.

DIAGNOSIS (di-ag-NO-sis): complete knowledge of patient's condition (pl. diagnoses).

DIALYSIS (di-AL-ih-sis): complete separation (-LYSIS) of wastes (urea) from the blood when the kidneys fail. See also HEMODIALYSIS and PERITONEAL DIALYSIS.

DIAPHRAGM (DI-ah-fram): muscle that separates the chest from the abdomen.

DIARRHEA (di-ah-RE-ah): Discharge of watery wastes from the COLON.

DIGESTIVE SYSTEM (di-JES-tiv SIS-tem): organs that bring food into the body and break it down to enter the bloodstream or eliminate it through the rectum and anus.

DILATION (di-LA-shun): widening, dilatation.

DILATION AND CURETTAGE (di-LA-shun and kur-eh-TAJ): widening of the cervix and scraping (curettage) of the inner lining of the uterus; *D&C.*

DISC (DISK): a piece of cartilage that is between each backbone.

DIURETICS (di-u-RET-iks): drugs that cause kidneys to allow more fluid (as urine) to leave the body; used to treat HYPERTENSION. DI- (from DIA-) means "complete" and UR- means urine.

DIVERTICULUM (di-ver-TIK-u-lum): a small pouch or sac created by a herniation of a mucous membrane lining (often in the intestines) (pl. diverticula).

DIVERTICULOSIS (di-ver-tik-u-LO-sis): abnormal condition of small pouches in the lining of the intestines.

DUODENAL (do-o-DE-nal): pertaining to the duodenum.

DUODENUM (do-o-DE-num): first part of the small intestine.

DYSENTERY (DIS-en-teh-re): abnormal, painful intestines.

DYSMENORRHEA (dis-men-o-RE-ah): painful menstrual flow.

DYSPEPSIA (dis-PEP-se-ah): painful (DYS-) digestion (-PEPSIA).

DYSPHASIA (dis-FA-zhah): difficult (impairment of) speech.

DYSPLASIA (dis-PLA-zhah): abnormality of development or formation of cells. Normal cells change in size, shape, and organization.

DYSPNEA (disp-NE-ah): painful (labored, difficult) breathing (-PNEA).

DYSURIA (dis-U-re-ah): painful or difficult urination.

EAR: organ that receives sound waves and transmits them to nerves leading to the brain.

EARDRUM (EAR-drum): membrane separating outer and middle part of the ear; tympanic membrane.

ECTOPIC PREGNANCY (ek-TOP-ik PREG-nan-se): development of the fetus in a place other than the uterus. The fallopian tubes are the most common ectopic site.

EDEMA (eh-DE-mah): swelling in tissues; often caused by retention (holding back) of fluid and salt by the kidneys.

ELECTROCARDIOGRAM (e-lek-tro-KAR-de-o-gram): record of the electricity in the heart.

ELECTROENCEPHALOGRAM (e-lek-tro-en-SEF-ah-lo-gram): record of the electricity in the brain.

EMBRYO (EM-bre-o): a new organism in the earliest stage of development. At the end of the second month of pregnancy, the developing baby is called a FETUS.

EMERGENCY MEDICINE (e-MER-jen-se MED-ih-sin): care of patients requiring immediate action.

EMPHYSEMA (em-fih-SE-mah): a lung disorder in which air becomes trapped in the air sacs and bronchioles, making breathing difficult. Marked by mucus accumulation and loss of elasticity in lung tissue.

ENCEPHALITIS (en-sef-ah-LI-tis): inflammation of the brain.

ENCEPHALOPATHY (en-sef-ah-LOP-ah-the): disease of the brain.

ENDOCRINE GLANDS (EN-do-krin glanz): organs that produce (secrete) hormones.

ENDOCRINE SYSTEM (EN-do krin SIS-tem): endocrine glands. Examples of endocrine glands are the pituitary, thyroid, and adrenal glands and the pancreas.

ENDOCRINOLOGIST (en-do-krih-NOL-o-jist): specialist in the study of endocrine glands and their disorders.

ENDOCRINOLOGY (en-do-krih-NOL-o-je): study of ENDOCRINE GLANDS.

ENDOMETRIOSIS (en-do-me-tre-O-sis): an abnormal condition in which tissue from the inner lining of the uterus is found outside the uterus, usually in the pelvic cavity.

ENDOMETRIUM (en-do-ME-tre-um): inner lining of the uterus.

ENDOSCOPE (EN-do-skop): instrument to view a hollow organ or body cavity; a tube fitted with a lens system that allows viewing in different directions.

ENDOSCOPY (en-DOS-ko-pe): process of viewing the inside of hollow organs or cavities by using an endoscope.

ENTERITIS (en-teh-RI-tis): inflammation of the small intestine.

EPIDERMIS (ep-i-DER-mis): the outer (EPI-) layer of the skin (-DERMIS).

EPIDURAL HEMATOMA (ep-ih-DUR-al he-mah-TO-mah): mass of blood above the dura mater (outermost layer of membranes surrounding the brain and spinal cord).

EPIGLOTTIS (ep-ih-GLOT-tis): flap of cartilage that covers the mouth of the trachea when swallowing occurs, so that food cannot enter the airway.

EPIGLOTTITIS (ep-ih-glo-TI-tis): inflammation of the EPIGLOTTIS.

EPILEPSY (ep-ih-LEP-se): abnormal electrical activity in the brain results in sudden, fleeting disturbances in nerve cell functioning. An attack of epilepsy is called a SEIZURE.

EPITHELIAL (ep-ih-THE-le-al): pertaining to skin cells. This term originally described cells upon (EPI-) the breast nipple (THELI-). Now, it indicates all cells lining the inner part of internal organs as well as covering the outside of the body.

ERYTHROCYTE (e-RITH-ro-sit): red blood cell.

ERYTHROCYTOSIS (e-rith-ro-si-TO-sis): abnormal condition (slight increase in numbers) of red blood cells.

ERYTHROMYCIN (e-rith-ro-MI-sin): an antibiotic that is produced from a red (ERYTHR/O) mold (-MYCIN).

ESOPHAGEAL (e-sof-ah-JE-al): pertaining to the esophagus.

EUSTACHIAN TUBE (u-STA-she-an tub): channel connecting the middle part of the ear with the throat.

EXCISION (ek-SIZH-un): to cut out; remove; resect.

EXOCRINE GLANDS (EK-so-krin glanz): produce (secrete) chemicals that leave the body through tubes (ducts). Examples are tear, sweat, and salivary glands.

EXOPHTHALMIC GOITER (ek-sof-THAL-mik GOY-ter): enlargement of the thyroid gland accompanied by high levels of thyroid hormone in the blood and protrusion of the eyeballs (EXOPHTHALMOS).

EXOPHTHALMOS (ek-sof-THAL-mos): abnormal protrusion of eyeballs; usually caused by HYPERTHYROIDISM.

EXTRAHEPATIC (eks-tra-heh-PAT-ik): pertaining to outside the liver.

EXTRAPULMONARY (eks-trah-PUL-mo-nah-re): outside the lungs.

EYE (i): organ that receives light waves and transmits them to the brain.

FALLOPIAN TUBES (fah-LO-pe-an tubz): two tubes that lead from the ovaries to the uterus. They transport egg cells to the uterus; also called uterine tubes.

FAMILY MEDICINE (FAM-i-le MED-ih-sin): primary care of all members of the family on a continuing basis.

FELLOWSHIP TRAINING (FEL-o-ship TRA-ning): postgraduate training for doctors in specialized fields. The training may include CLINICAL and RESEARCH (laboratory) work.

FEMALE REPRODUCTIVE SYSTEM (FE-mal re-pro-DUK-tiv SIS-tem): organs that produce (OVARY) and transport (FALLOPIAN TUBES) egg cells and secrete female hormones (ESTROGEN and PROGESTERONE). The system includes the UTERUS, where the embryo and fetus grow.

FEMUR (FE-mer): thigh bone.

FETUS (FE-tus): unborn infant in the uterus after the second month of pregnancy.

FIBRILLATION (fih-brih-LA-shun): rapid, irregular, involuntary muscular contraction. Atrial and ventricular fibrillation are cardiac (heart) ARRHYTHMIAS.

FIBROIDS (FI-broydz): benign growth of muscle tissue in the uterus.

FIBULA (FIB-u-lah): smaller lower leg bone.

FIXATION (fik-SA-shun): the act of holding, sewing, or fastening a part in a fixed position.

FLUTTER (FLUT-er): rapid, but regular abnormal heart muscle contraction. Atrial and ventricular flutter are heart ARRHYTHMIAS.

FRACTURE (FRAK-tur): breaking of a bone.

FRONTAL (FRUN-tal): pertaining to the front; anterior.

FRONTAL PLANE (FRUN-tal plan): an imaginary line that divides an organ or the body into a front and back portion; coronal plane.

GALLBLADDER (GAL-bla-der): sac below the liver; stores bile and delivers it to the small intestine.

GANGLION (GANG-le-on): benign cyst near a joint (wrist); also, a group of nerve cells; pl. ganglia (GANG-le-ah).

GASTRALGIA (gas-TRAL-jah): stomach pain.

GASTRECTOMY (gas-TREK-to-me): excision (removal) of the stomach.

GASTRIC (GAS-trik): pertaining to the stomach.

GASTRITIS (gas-TRI-tis): inflammation of the stomach.

GASTROENTERITIS (gas-tro-en-teh-RI-tis): inflammation of the stomach and intestines.

GASTROENTEROLOGIST (gas-tro-en-ter-OL-o-jist): specialist in the treatment of stomach and intestinal disorders.

GASTROENTEROLOGY (gas-tro-en-ter-OL-o-je): study of the stomach and intestines.

GASTROJEJUNOSTOMY (gas-tro-jeh-ju-NOS-to-me): new surgical opening between the stomach and the jejunum (second part of the small intestine).

GASTROSCOPE (GAS-tro-skop): instrument to view the stomach. It is passed down the throat and esophagus into the stomach.

GASTROSCOPY (gas-TROS-ko-pe): visual examination of the stomach.

GASTROTOMY (gas-TROT-o-me): incision of the stomach.

GERIATRICIAN (jer-e-ah-TRISH-an): specialist in the treatment of diseases of old age.

GERIATRICS (jer-e-AH-triks): treatment of disorders of old age.

GLAND: a group of cells that secrete chemicals to the outside of the body (EXOCRINE GLANDS) or directly into the bloodstream (ENDOCRINE GLANDS).

GLAUCOMA (glaw-KO-mah): increase of fluid pressure within the eye; fluid is formed more rapidly than it is removed. The increased pressure damages sensitive cells in the back of the eye and vision is disturbed.

GLIOBLASTOMA (gli-o-blas-TO-mah): a malignant brain tumor composed of immature (-BLAST) neuroglial (supportive nervous tissue) cells.

GLYCOSURIA (gli-ko-SU-re-ah): abnormal condition of sugar in the urine.

GOITER (GOY-ter): enlargement of the thyroid gland.

GOUTY ARTHRITIS (gowti arth-RI-tis): deposits of uric acid crystals in joints and other tissues and causing swelling and inflammation of joints. Also called gout.

GRAVES DISEASE (gravs dih-ZEZ): see HYPERTHYROIDISM.

GYNECOLOGIST (gi-neh-KOL-o-jist): specialist in medical and surgical treatment of female disorders.

GYNECOLOGY (gi-neh-KOL-o-je): study of female disorders.

HAIR FOLLICLE (hahr FOL-ih-kl): a pouch-like depression in the skin in which a hair develops.

HAIR ROOT (hahr root): part of the hair from which growth occurs.

HEART (hart): hollow, muscular organ in the chest; pumps blood throughout the body.

HEMATEMESIS (he-mah-TEM-eh-sis): vomiting (-EMESIS) blood (HEMAT/O).

HEMATOLOGIST (he-mah-TOL-o-jist): specialist in blood and blood disorders.

HEMATOMA (he-mah-TO-mah): mass or collection of blood under the skin; commonly called a bruise or black-and-blue mark.

HEMATURIA (he-mah-TUR-e-ah): abnormal condition of blood in the urine.

HEMIPLEGIA (hem-ih-PLE-jah): paralysis of one side of the body.

HEMODIALYSIS (he-mo-di-AL-ih-sis): use of a kidney machine to filter blood to remove waste materials, such as urea. Blood leaves the body, enters the machine, and is carried back to the body through a catheter (tube).

HEMOGLOBIN (HE-mo-glo-bin): oxygen-carrying protein found in red blood cells.

HEMOPTYSIS (he-MOP-tih-sis): spitting up (-PTYSIS) blood (HEM/O).

HEMORRHAGE (HEM-or-ij): bursting forth of blood.

HEMOTHORAX (he-mo-THOR-aks): collection of blood in the chest (pleural cavity).

HEPATIC (heh-PAT-ik): pertaining to the liver.

HEPATITIS (hep-ah-TI-tis): inflammation of the liver. Viral hepatitis is an acute infectious disease caused by at least three different viruses: hepatitis A, B, and C viruses.

HEPATOMA (hep-ah-TO-mah): tumor (malignant) of the liver; hepatocellular carcinoma.

HEPATOMEGALY (hep-ah-to-MEG-ah-le): enlargement of the liver.

HERNIA (HER-ne-ah): bulge or protrusion of an organ or part of an organ through the wall of the cavity that usually contains it. In an INGUINAL hernia, part of the wall of the abdomen weakens and the intestine bulges out or into the SCROTAL sac (in males).

HIATAL HERNIA (hi-A-tal HER-ne-ah): upward protrusion of the wall of the stomach into the lower part of the esophagus.

HIV: see HUMAN IMMUNODEFICIENCY VIRUS.

HODGKIN DISEASE (HOJ-kin di-ZEZ): malignant tumor of lymph nodes.

HORMONE (HOR-mon): chemical made by a gland and sent directly into the bloodstream, not to the outside of the body. ENDOCRINE GLANDS produce hormones.

HUMAN IMMUNODEFICIENCY VIRUS (U-man im-u-no-deh-FISH-en-se VI-rus): infects white blood cells (T cell lymphocytes) causing damage to the patient's immune system. HIV is the cause of AIDS.

HUMERUS (HU-mer-us): upper arm bone.

HYDROCELE (HI-dro-sel): swelling of the SCROTUM caused by a collection of fluid within the outermost covering of the TESTIS.

HYPERGLYCEMIA (hi-per-gli-SE-me-ah): higher than normal levels of sugar in the blood.

HYPERPARATHYROIDISM (hi-per-par-ah-THI-royd-ism): higher than normal levels of parathyroid hormone in the blood.

HYPERTENSION (hi-per-TEN-shun): high blood pressure. *Essential hypertension* has no known cause, but contributing factors are age, obesity, smoking, and heredity. *Secondary hypertension* is a symptom of other disorders such as kidney disease.

HYPERTHYROIDISM (hi-per-THI-royd-izm): excessive activity of the thyroid gland.

HYPERTROPHY (hi-PER-tro-fe): enlargement or overgrowth of an organ or part of the body due to an increase in size of individual cells.

HYPODERMIC (hi-po-DER-mik): pertaining to under or below the skin.

HYPOGLYCEMIA (hi-po-gli-SE-me-ah): lower than normal blood sugar levels.

HYPOPHYSEAL (hi-po-FIZ-e-al): pertaining to the pituitary gland.

HYPOPITUITARISM (hi-po-pi-TU-ih-tah-rizm): decrease or stoppage of hormonal secretion by the pituitary gland.

HYPOTENSIVE (hi-po-TEN-siv): pertaining to low blood pressure or to a person with abnormally low blood pressure.

HYPOTHYROIDISM (hi-po-THI-royd-izm): lower than normal activity of the thyroid gland.

HYSTERECTOMY (his-teh-REK-to-me): excision of the uterus, either through the abdominal wall (abdominal hysterectomy) or through the vagina (vaginal hysterectomy).

IATROGENIC (i-ah-tro-JEN-ik): pertaining to a patient's abnormal condition that results unexpectedly from a specific treatment.

ILEOSTOMY (il-e-OS-to-me): new opening of the ileum (third part of the small intestine) to the outside of the body.

ILEUM (IL-e-um): third part of the small intestine.

ILIUM (IL-e-um): side, high portion of the hip bone (pelvis).

INCISION (in-SIZH-un): cutting into the body or into an organ.

INFARCTION (in-FARK-shun): area of dead tissue caused by decreased blood flow to that part of the body.

INFECTIOUS DISEASE SPECIALIST (in-FEK-shus dih-ZEZ SPESH-ah-list): physician who treats disorders caused and spread by microorganisms such as bacteria.

INFILTRATE (IN-fil-trat): material that accumulates in an organ; often describes solid material and fluid collection in the lungs.

INFLAMMATORY BOWEL DISEASE (in-FLAM-ah-to-re BOW-el di-ZEZ): disorder of the small and large intestines marked by bouts of diarrhea, abdominal cramping, and fever; includes CROHN DISEASE and ULCERATIVE COLITIS.

INGUINAL (ING-gwi-nal): pertaining to the groin; area where the legs meet the body.

INSULIN (IN-su-lin): hormone produced by the pancreas and released into the bloodstream. Insulin allows sugar to leave the blood and enter body cells.

INTERNAL MEDICINE (in-TER-nal MED-ih-sin): branch of medicine specializing in the diagnosis of disorders and treatment with drugs.

INTERVERTEBRAL (in-ter-VER-teh-bral): pertaining to lying between two backbones. A disk (disc) is an intervertebral structure.

INTRA-ABDOMINAL (in-trah-ab-DOM-ih-nal): pertaining to within the abdomen.

INTRAUTERINE (in-trah-U-ter-in): pertaining to within the uterus.

INTRAVENOUS (in-trah-VE-nus): pertaining to within a vein.

INTRAVENOUS PYELOGRAM (in-trah-VEN-nus PI-eh-lo-gram): x-ray record of the kidney (PYEL/O means renal pelvis) after contrast is injected into a vein.

IRIS (I-ris): colored (pigmented) portion of the eye.

ISCHEMIA (is-KE-me-ah): deficiency of blood flow to a part of the body, caused by narrowing or obstruction of blood vessels.

JAUNDICE (JAWN-dis): orange-yellow coloration of the skin and other tissues. A symptom caused by accumulation of BILIRUBIN (pigment) in the blood.

JEJUNUM (jeh-JE-num): second part of the small intestine.

JOINT (joynt): space where two or more bones come together (articulate).

KIDNEY (KID-ne): one of two organs behind the abdomen that produces urine by filtering wastes from the blood.

LAPAROSCOPY (lap-ah-ROS-ko-pe): visual examination of the abdomen. A small incision is made near the navel, and an instrument is inserted to view abdominal organs.

LAPAROTOMY (lap-ah-ROT-o-me): incision of the abdomen. A surgeon makes a large incision across the abdomen to examine and operate on its organs.

LARGE INTESTINE (larj-in-TES-tin): part of the intestine that receives undigested material from the small intestine and transports out of the body; COLON.

LARYNGEAL (lah-rin-JE-al): pertaining to the larynx (voice box).

LARYNGECTOMY (lah-rin-JEK-to-me): removal of the larynx (voice box).

LARYNGITIS (lah-rin-JI-tis): inflammation of the larynx.

LARYNGOTRACHEITIS (lah-ring-o-tra-ke-I-tis): inflammation of the larynx and the trachea (windpipe).

LARYNX (LAR-inks): voice box; located at the top of the trachea and containing vocal cords.

LATERAL (LAT-er-al): pertaining to the side.

LEIOMYOMA (li-o-mi-O-mah): a benign tumor derived from smooth (involuntary) muscle and most often of the uterus (leiomyoma uteri).

LENS (lenz): structure behind the pupil of the eye; bends light rays so that they are properly focused on the RETINA at the back of the eye.

LESION (LE-zhun): any damage to a part of the body, caused by disease or trauma.

LEUKEMIA (lu-KE-me-ah): excess numbers of malignant white blood cells in blood and bone marrow.

LIGAMENT (LIG-ah-ment): connective tissue that joins bones to other bones.

LIGAMENTOUS (lig-ah-MEN-tus): pertaining to a LIGAMENT.

LITHOTRIPSY (lith-o-TRIP-se): process of crushing a stone in the urinary tract using ultrasonic vibrations.

LIVER (LIV-er): organ in the right upper quadrant of the abdomen; produces BILE, stores sugar, and produces blood clotting proteins.

LOBE (lob): part of an organ, especially of the brain, lungs, or glands.

LUMBAR (LUM-bar): pertaining to the loins; part of the back and sides between the chest and the hip.

LUMBAR REGION (LUM-bar RE-jin): pertaining to the backbones that lie between the thoracic (chest) and sacral (lower back) vertebrae.

LUMBAR VERTEBRA (LUM-bar VER-teh-brah): a backbone in the region between the chest and lower back.

LUNG (lung): one of two paired organs in the chest through which oxygen enters and carbon dioxide leaves the body.

LUNG CAPILLARIES (lung KAP-ih-lar-ez): tiny blood vessels surrounding lung tissue and through which gases pass into and out of the bloodstream.

LYMPH (limf): clear fluid that is found in lymph vessels and produced from fluid surrounding cells. Lymph contains white blood cells (lymphocytes) that fight disease.

LYMPHADENECTOMY (limf-ah-deh-NEK-to-me): removal of LYMPH NODES.

LYMPH NODE (limf nod): stationary collection of lymph cells; found all over the body.

LYMPHADENOPATHY (lim-fad-eh-NOP-ah-the): disease of lymph nodes (glands).

LYMPHANGIOGRAM (lim-FAN-je-o-gram): x-ray record of lymph vessels after contrast is injected into soft tissue of the foot.

LYMPHATIC VESSELS (lim-FAT-ik VES-elz): tubes that carry lymph from tissues to the bloodstream (into a vein in the neck region); lymph vessels.

LYMPHOCYTE (LIMF-o-sit): white blood cell that is found within lymph and lymph nodes. T cells and B cells are types of lymphocytes.

LYMPHOPOIESIS (limf-o-POY-e-sis): formation of lymph.

MAGNETIC RESONANCE IMAGING (mag-NET-ik REZ-o-nans IM-aj-ing): image of the body using magnetic and radio waves. Organs are seen in three planes: frontal (front to back), sagittal (side to side), and transverse (cross-section). Called *MRI*.

MALE REPRODUCTIVE SYSTEM (mal re-pro-DUK-tiv SIS-tem): organs that produce sperm cells and male hormones.

MALIGNANT (mah-LIG-nant): tending to become progressively worse; describes cancerous tumors that invade and spread to distant organs.

MAMMARY (MAM-er-e): pertaining to the breast.

MAMMOGRAM (MAM-o-gram): x-ray record of the breast.

MAMMOGRAPHY (mam-OG-rah-fe): process of x-ray recording of the breast.

MAMMOPLASTY (MAM-o-plas-te): surgical repair (reconstruction) of the breast.

MASTECTOMY (mas-TEK-to-me): removal (excision) of the breast.

MEDIASTINAL (me-de-ah-STI-nal): pertaining to the MEDIASTINUM.

MEDIASTINUM (me-de-ah-STI-num): space between the lungs in the chest; contains the heart, large blood vessels, trachea, esophagus, thymus gland, and lymph nodes.

MEDULLARY (MEH-DU-lar-e): pertaining to the inner, or soft part of an organ.

MEDULLA OBLONGATA (meh-DUL-ah ob-lon-GA-tah): lower part of the brain near the spinal cord; controls breathing and heartbeat.

MELANOMA (meh-lah-NO-mah): malignant tumor arising from pigmented cells (melanocytes) in the skin; usually developing from a NEVUS (mole).

MENINGITIS (men-in-JI-tis): inflammation of the meninges (membranes around the brain and spinal cord).

MENORRHAGIA (men-o-RA-je-ah): excessive bleeding from the uterus during the time of MENSTRUATION.

MENORRHEA (men-o-RE-ah): normal discharge of blood and tissue from the uterine lining during MENSTRUATION.

MENSES (MEN-sez): menstruation; menstrual period.

MENSTRUATION (men-stru-A-shun): breakdown of the lining of the uterus that occurs every four weeks during the active reproductive period of a female.

METACARPALS (met-ah-KAR-palz): bones of the hand between the wrist bones (carpals) and the finger bones (phalanges).

METASTASIS (meh-TAS-tah-sis): spread of a cancerous tumor to a distant organ or location; literally means change (META-) of place (-STASIS).

METATARSALS (meh-tah-TAR-sels): foot bones.

MIGRAINE (MI-gran): attack of headache; usually on one side of the head, caused by changes in blood vessel size and accompanied by nausea, vomiting, and sensitivity to light (photophobia). From the French word *migraine,* meaning "severe head pain."

MOUTH (mowth): the opening that forms the beginning of the digestive system.

MONOCYTE (MON-o-sit): white blood cell with one large nucleus.

MONONUCLEOSIS (mon-o-nu-kle-O-sis): an acute infectious disease with excess MONOCYTES in the blood. Caused by the Epstein-Barr virus and transmitted by direct oral (mouth) contact.

MRI: see MAGNETIC RESONANCE IMAGING.

MULTIPLE SCLEROSIS (MUL-tih-pul skeh-RO-sis): chronic neurological disease in which there are patches of loss of MYELIN SHEATH (covering neurons) throughout the brain and spinal cord. Weakness, abnormal sensations, incoordination, and speech and visual disturbances are symptoms.

MUSCLE (MUS-el): connective tissue that contracts to make movement possible.

MUSCULAR (MUS-ku-lar): pertaining to muscles.

MUSCULAR DYSTROPHY (MUS-ku-lar DIS-tro-fe): group of degenerative muscle diseases that cause crippling because muscles are gradually weakened and eventually ATROPHY (shrink).

MUSCULOSKELETAL SYSTEM (mus-ku-lo-SKEL-e-tal SYS-tem): organs that support the body and allow it to move; muscles, bones, joints, and connective tissues.

MYALGIA (mi-AL-jah): pain in a muscle or muscles.

MYELIN SHEATH (MI-eh-lin sheat): fatty covering around part (axon) of some nerve fibers. It insulates and speeds the conduction of nerve impulses.

MYELODYSPLASIA (mi-eh-lo-dis-PLA-ze-ah): abnormal development of bone marrow; a premalignant condition leading to leukemia.

MYELOGRAM (MI-eh-lo-gram): x-ray record of the spinal cord after contrast is injected within the membranes surrounding the spinal cord in the lumbar area of the back.

MYELOGRAPHY (mi-eh-LOG-ra-fe): process of recording the spinal cord after injection of contrast material.

MYOCARDIAL (mi-o-KAR-de-al): pertaining to the muscle of the heart.

MYOCARDIAL INFARCTION (mi-o-KAR-de-al in-FARK-shun): area of dead tissue in heart muscle; also known as a heart attack or an *MI*.

MYOMA (mi-O-mah): tumor (benign) of muscle.

MYOSARCOMA (mi-o-sar-KO-mah): tumor (malignant) of muscle. SARC- means "flesh," indicating that the tumor is of connective or "fleshy" tissue origin.

MYOSITIS (mi-o-SI-tis): inflammation of a muscle.

MYRINGOTOMY (mir-in-GOT-o-me): incision of the eardrum.

NASAL (NA-zel): pertaining to the nose.

NAUSEA (NAW-se-ah): an unpleasant sensation in the upper abdomen, often leading to vomiting. The term comes from the Greek *nausia*, meaning "sea sickness."

NECROSIS (neh-KRO-sis): death of cells.

NECROTIC (neh-KRO-tik): pertaining to death of cells.

NEONATAL (ne-o-NA-tal): pertaining to new birth; the period of first four weeks after birth.

NEOPLASM (NE-o-plazm): any new growth of tissue; a tumor.

NEOPLASTIC (ne-o-PLAS-tik): pertaining to a new growth or NEOPLASM.

NEPHRECTOMY (neh-FREK-to-me): removal (excision) of a kidney.

NEPHRITIS (neh-FRI-tis): inflammation of the kidneys.

NEPHROLITHIASIS (neh-fro-lih-THI-ah-sis): condition of kidney stones.

NEPHROLOGIST (neh-FROL-o-jist): specialist in diagnosis and treatment of kidney diseases.

NEPHROLOGY (neh-FROL-o-je): study of the kidney and its diseases.

NEPHROPATHY (neh-FROP-ah-the): disease of the kidney.

NEPHROSIS (neh-FRO-sis): abnormal condition of the kidney. This condition is often associated with a deterioration of kidney tubules.

NEPHROSTOMY (neh-FROS-to-me): opening from the kidney to the outside of the body.

NERVOUS SYSTEM (NER-vus SIS-tem): organs (brain, spinal cord, and nerves) that transmit electrical messages throughout the body.

NEURAL (NU-ral): pertaining to nerves.

NEURALGIA (nu-RAL-jah): nerve pain.

NEURITIS (nu-RI-tis): inflammation of a nerve.

NEUROGLIAL CELLS (nu-ro-GLE-al selz): supporting structure of nervous tissue in the central nervous system, such as the brain. Examples are astrocytes, microglial, and oligodendroglial cells. These cells are often the source of brain tumors.

NEUROLOGIST (nu-ROL-o-jist): specialist in the diagnosis and treatment of nervous disorders.

NEUROLOGY (nu-ROL-o-je): study of the nervous system and nerve disorders.

NEUROPATHY (nu-ROP-ah-the): disease of nervous tissue.

NEUROSURGEON (nu-ro-SUR-jin): physician who operates on the organs of the nervous system (brain, spinal cord, and nerves).

NEUROTOMY (nu-ROT-o-me): incision of a nerve.

NEVUS (NE-vus): pigmented lesion on the skin; a mole.

NOCTURIA (nok-TU-re-ah): excessive urination at night.

NOSE (noz): structure that is the organ of smell and permits air to enter and leave the body.

NOSOCOMIAL (nos-o-KO-me-al): pertaining to or originating in a hospital. A nosocomial infection is acquired during hospitalization.

OBSTETRIC (ob-STEH-TRIK): pertaining to pregnancy, labor, and delivery of an infant.

OBSTETRICIAN (ob-steh-TRISH-un): specialist in the delivery of a baby and care of the mother during pregnancy and labor.

OCULAR (OK-u-lar): pertaining to the eye.

ONCOGENIC (ong-ko-JEN-ik): pertaining to producing (GEN) tumors.

ONCOLOGIST (ong-KOL-o-jist): physician specializing in the study and treatment of tumors.

ONCOLOGY (ong-KOL-o-je): study of tumors.

OOPHORECTOMY (o-of-o-REK-to me): removal (excision) of an ovary or ovaries.

OOPHORITIS (o-of-o-RI-tis): inflammation of an ovary.

OPHTHALMOLOGIST (of-thal-MOL-o-jist): specialist in the study of the eye and treatment of eye disorders.

OPHTHALMOLOGY (of-thal-MOL-o-je): study of the eye; diagnosis and treatment of eye disorders.

OPTIC NERVE (OP-tik nerv): nerve in the back of the eye that transmits light waves to the brain.

OPTICIAN (op-TISH-an): non-medical specialist in providing eye glasses by filling prescriptions.

OPTOMETRIST (op-TOM-eh-trist): non-medical specialist trained to examine and test eyes and prescribe corrective lenses.

ORAL (OR-al): pertaining to the mouth.

ORCHIDECTOMY (or-kih-DEK-to-me): removal (excision) of a testicle or testicles.

ORCHIECTOMY (or-ke-EK-to-me): removal (excision) of a testicle or testicles.

ORCHIOPEXY (or-ke-o-PEK-se): surgical fixation of the testicle (testis) into its proper location within the scrotum. This surgery corrects CRYPTORCHISM.

ORCHITIS (or-KI-tis): inflammation of a testicle.

ORGAN (OR-gan): an independent part of the body, composed of different tissues working together to do a specific job.

ORTHOPEDIST (or-tho-PE-dist): specialist in surgical correction of musculo-skeletal disorders. This physician was originally concerned with straightening (ORTH/O) bones in the legs of deformed children (PED/O).

OSTEITIS (os-te-I-tis): inflammation of a bone.

OSTEOARTHRITIS (os-te-o-ar-THRI-tis): inflammation of bones and joints. This is a disease of older people, marked by stiffness, pain, and degeneration of joints.

OSTEOMA (os-te-O-mah): tumor (benign) of bone.

OSTEOMYELITIS (os-te-o-mi-eh-LI-tis): inflammation of bone and bone marrow. This condition is caused by a bacterial infection.

OSTEOPOROSIS (os-te-o-po-RO-sis): decrease in bone mass with formation of pores or spaces in normally mineralized bone tissue.

OTALGIA (o-TAL-jah): pain in an ear.

OTITIS (o-TI-tis): inflammation of an ear.

OTOLARYNGOLOGIST (o-to-lah-rin-GOL-o-jist): specialist in treatment of diseases of the ear, nose, and throat.

OVARIAN (o-VAR-e-an): pertaining to an OVARY or ovaries.

OVARIAN CANCER (o-VAR-e-an KAN-ser): malignant condition of the ovaries.

OVARIAN CYST (o-VAR-e-an sist): a sac containing fluid or semi-solid material in or on the ovary.

OVARY (O-vah-re): one of two organs in the female abdomen that produces egg cells and female hormones.

OVUM (O-vum): an egg cell; pl. ova (o-VAH).

OXYGEN (OK-si-jen): a colorless, odorless gas that is essential to sustaining life.

PANCREAS (PAN-kre-us): gland that produces digestive juices (exocrine function), and the hormone, INSULIN (endocrine function).

PANCREATECTOMY (pan-kre-ah-TEK-to-me): removal of the pancreas.

PANCREATITIS (pan-kre-ah-TI-tis): inflammation of the pancreas.

PARALYSIS (pah-RAL-ih-sis): loss or impairment of movement in a part of the body.

PARAPLEGIA (par-ah-PLE-jah): impairment or loss of movement in the lower part of the body, primarily the legs and in some cases bowel and bladder function.

PARATHYROID GLANDS (par-ah-THI-royd glanz): four endocrine glands behind the thyroid gland. These glands are concerned with maintaining the proper levels of calcium in the blood and bones.

PATELLA (pah-TEL-ah): knee cap.

PATHOLOGIST (pah-THOL-o-jist): specialist in the study of disease, by microscopic examination of tissues and cells and autopsy examination.

PATHOLOGY (pah-THOL-o-je): study of disease.

PEDIATRICIAN (pe-de-ah-TRISH-un): specialist in treatment of childhood diseases.

PEDIATRICS (pe-de-AT-riks): branch of medicine specializing in treatment of children.

PELVIC (PEL-vik): pertaining to the hip bone (pelvis) or the region of the hip.

PELVIC CAVITY (PEL-vik KAV-ih-te): space contained within the hip bone (front and sides) and the lower part of the backbone (sacrum and coccyx).

PELVIC INFLAMMATORY DISEASE (PEL-vik in-FLAM-ah-to-re di-ZEZ): inflammation in the pelvic region; usually inflammation of the fallopian tubes.

PELVIS (PEL-vis): hip bone. The pelvis is composed of the ilium (upper portion), ischium (lower portion), and the pubis (front portion).

PENICILLIN (pen-in-SIL-in): substance, derived from certain molds, that can destroy bacteria; an ANTIBIOTIC.

PENIS (PE-nis): external male organ containing the urethra, through which both urine and semen (sperm cells and fluid) leave the body.

PEPTIC ULCER (PEP-tik UL-ser): sore (lesion) of the mucous membrane lining the first part of the small intestine (duodenum) or lining the stomach.

PERCUTANEOUS (per-ku-TAN-e-us): pertaining to through the skin.

PERIANAL (per-e-A-nal): pertaining to surrounding the ANUS.

PERIOSTEUM (per-e-OS-te-um): membrane that surrounds bone.

PERITONEAL (per-ih-to-NE-al): pertaining to the PERITONEUM.

PERITONEAL DIALYSIS (per-i-to-NE-al di-AL-ih-sis): process of removing wastes from the blood by introducing a special fluid into the abdomen. The wastes pass into the fluid from the bloodstream, and then the fluid is drained from the body.

PERITONEUM (per-ih-to-NE-um): membrane that surrounds the abdomen and holds the abdominal organs in place.

PHALANGES (fah-LAN-jez): finger and toe bones.

PHARYNGEAL (fah-rin-JE-al): pertaining to the pharynx (throat).

PHARYNGITIS (fah-rin-JI-tis): inflammation of the pharynx (throat).

PHARYNX (FAR-inks): organ behind the mouth that receives swallowed food and delivers it into the esophagus. The pharynx (throat) also receives air from the nose and passes it to the trachea (windpipe).

PHLEBITIS (fleh-BI-tis): inflammation of a vein.

PHLEBOTOMY (fleh-BOT-o-me): incision of a vein.

PHRENIC (FREH-nik): pertaining to the DIAPHRAGM.

PHYSICAL MEDICINE AND REHABILITATION (FIZ-e-kal MED-i-sin and re-ha-bil-i-TA-shun): field of medicine that specializes in restoring the function of the body after illness.

PINEAL GLAND (pi-NE-al gland): small endocrine gland within the brain; secretes a hormone, melatonin, whose exact function is unclear. In lower animals it is a receptor for light.

PITUITARY GLAND (pi-TU-ih-tar-e gland): organ at the base of the brain that secretes hormones. These hormones enter the blood to regulate other organs and other endocrine glands.

PLATELET (PLAT-let): cell in the blood that aids clotting; thrombocyte.

PLEURA (PLOO-rah): double membrane that surrounds the lungs.

PLEURAL EFFUSION (PLOO-ral e-FU-zhun): collection of fluid between the double membrane surrounding the lungs.

PLEURISY (PLOO-ih-se): inflammation of the PLEURA.

PLEURITIS (ploo-RI-tis): inflammation of the PLEURA.

PNEUMOCONIOSIS (noo-mo-ko-ne-O-sis): group of lung diseases resulting from inhalation of particles of dust such as coal, with permanent deposition of such particles in the lung.

PNEUMONIA (noo-MO-ne-ah): abnormal condition of the lungs, marked by inflammation and collection of material within the air sacs of the lungs.

PNEUMONITIS (noo-mo-NI-tis): inflammation of a lung or lungs.

PNEUMONECTOMY (noo-mo-NEK-to-me): removal of a lung.

PNEUMOTHORAX (noo-mo-THO-raks): abnormal accumulation of air in the space between the pleura.

POLYCYTHEMIA (pol-e-si-THE-me-ah): increase in red blood cells. One form is polycythemia vera, in which the bone marrow produces an excess of erythrocytes.

POLYDIPSIA (pol-e-DIP-se-ah): excessive thirst.

POLYP (POL-ip): a growth or mass (benign) protruding from a mucous membrane, and hemoglobin level is elevated.

POLYURIA (pol-e-UR-e-ah): excessive urination.

POST MORTEM (post MOR-tem): after death.

POST PARTUM (post PAR-tum): after birth.

POSTERIOR (pos-TER-e-or): located in the back portion of a structure or of the body.

PRECANCEROUS (pre-KAN-ser-us): pertaining to a condition that may come before a cancer; a condition that tends to become malignant.

PRENATAL (pre-NA-tal): pertaining to before birth.

PROCTOLOGIST (prok-TOL-o-jist): physician who specializes in the study of the anus and rectum.

PROCTOSCOPY (prok-TOS-ko-pe): inspection of the anus and rectum with a proctoscope (ENDOSCOPE); often done prior to rectal surgery.

PROGNOSIS (prog-NO-sis): forecast as to the probable outcome of an illness or treatment; literally, before (PRO-) knowledge (-GNOSIS).

PROLAPSE (pro-LAPS): falling down, drooping of a part of the body; literally, a sliding (-LAPSE) forward (PRO-).

PROSTATE GLAND (PROS-tat gland): male gland that surrounds the base of the urinary bladder. It produces fluid that leaves the body with sperm cells.

PROSTATECTOMY (pros-tah-TEK-to-me): removal of the prostate gland.

PROSTATIC (pros-TAH-tik): pertaining to the prostate gland.

PROSTATIC CARCINOMA (pros-TAH-tik kar-si-NO-mah): malignant tumor arising from the PROSTATE GLAND.

PROSTATIC HYPERPLASIA (pros-TAH-tik hi-per-PLA-zhah): abnormal increase in growth (benign) of the prostate gland.

PROSTHESIS (pros-THE-sis): artificial substitute for a missing part of the body; literally, to place (-THESIS) before (PROS-).

PROTEINURIA (pro-en-U-re-ah): abnormal condition of protein in the urine (albuminuria).

PSYCHIATRIST (si-KI-ah-trist): specialist in treatment of the mind and mental disorders.

PSYCHIATRY (si-KI-ah-tre): treatment (IATR/O) of disorders of the mind (PSYCH/O).

PSYCHOLOGY (si-KOL-o-je): study of the mind; especially in relation to human behavior.

PSYCHOSIS (si-KO-sis): abnormal condition of the mind; serious mental disorder that involves loss of normal perception of reality; pl. psychoses (si-KO-sez).

PULMONARY (PUL-mo-ner-e): pertaining to the lungs.

PULMONARY CIRCULATION (PUL-mo-ner-e ser-ku-LA-shun): passage of blood from the heart to the lungs and back to the heart.

PULMONARY EDEMA (PUL-mo-ner-e eh-DE-mah): abnormal collection of fluid in the lung (within the air sacs of the lung).

PULMONARY SPECIALIST (PUL-mo-ner-e SPESH-ah-list): physician trained to treat lung disorders.

PUPIL (PU-pil): black center of the eye through which light enters.

PYELITIS (pi-eh-LI-tis): inflammation of the renal pelvis (central section of the kidney).

RADIATION ONCOLOGIST (ra-de-A-shun ong-KOL-o-jist): physician trained in treatment of disease (cancer) using high-energy x-rays or other particles.

RADIOLOGIST (ra-de-OL-o-jist): physician trained in the use of x-rays to diagnose illness; also includes ultrasound and magnetic resonance imaging techniques.

RADIOLOGY (ra-de-OL-o-je): science of using x-rays in the diagnosis of disease.

RADIOTHERAPY (ra-de-o-THER-ah-pe): treatment of disease (cancer) using high-energy particles, such as x-rays and protons.

RADIUS (RA-de-us): one of two lower arm bones; on the thumb side of the hand.

RECTAL RESECTION (REK-tal re-SEK-shun): excision (resection) of the RECTUM.

RECTOCELE (REK-to-sel): hernia (protrusion) of the rectum into the vagina.

RECTUM (REK-tum): end of the colon; delivers wastes (feces) to the anus for elimination.

RELAPSE (re-LAPS): return of disease after its apparent termination.

REMISSION (re-MISH-un): lessening of symptoms of a disease.

RENAL (RE-nal): pertaining to the kidney.

RENAL FAILURE (RE-nal FAL-ur): kidneys no longer function.

RENAL PELVIS (RE-nal PEL-vis): central section of the kidney, where urine collects.

RESEARCH (RE-surch): laboratory investigation of a medical problem.

RESECTION (re-SEK-shun): removal of an organ or a structure.

RESIDENCY TRAINING (RES-i-den-se TRAY-ning): period of hospital work involving care of patients after completion of four years of medical school.

RESPIRATORY SYSTEM (RES-pir-ah-tor-e SIS-tem): organs that control breathing, allowing air to enter and leave the body.

RETINA (RET-ih-nah): layer of sensitive cells at the back of the eye. Light is focused on the retina and then is transmitted to the optic nerve, which leads to the brain.

RETINOPATHY (reh-tih-NOP-ah-the): disease of the RETINA.

RETROGASTRIC (reh-tro-GAS-trik): pertaining to behind the stomach.

RETROPERITONEAL (reh-tro-per-ih-to-NE-al): pertaining to behind the PERITONEUM.

RHEUMATOID ARTHRITIS (ROO-mah-toyd arth-RI-tis): chronic inflammatory disease of joints and connective tissue leading to deformed joints.

RHEUMATOLOGIST (roo-mah-TOL-o-jist): specialist in treatment of diseases of connective tissues, especially joints. RHEUMAT/O comes from the Greek *rheuma,* meaning "that which flows, as a stream or a river." Inflammatory disorders of joints are often marked by a collection of fluid in joint spaces.

RHEUMATOLOGY (roo-mah-TOL-o-je): branch of medicine dealing with inflammation, degeneration, or chemical changes in connective tissues, such as joints and muscles. Pain, stiffness, or limitation of motion are often characteristics of rheumatologic disorders.

RHINITIS (ri-NI-tis): inflammation of the nose.

RHINOPLASTY (RI-no-plas-te): surgical repair of the nose.

RHINORRHEA (ri-no-RE-ah): discharge from the nose.

RHINOTOMY (ri-NOT-o-me): incision of the nose.

RIB (rib): one of twelve paired bones surrounding the chest. Seven ribs (true ribs) attach directly to the breastbone, three (false ribs) attach to the seventh rib, and two (floating ribs) are not attached at all.

SACRAL (SA-kral): pertaining to the SACRUM.

SACRAL REGION (SA-kral RE-jin): five fused bones in the lower back, below the lumbar bones and wedged between two parts of the hip (ilium).

SACRUM (SA-krum): triangular bone in the lower back; below the lumbar bones and formed by five fused bones.

SAGITTAL PLANE (SAJ-ih-tal plan): an imaginary line that divides an organ or the body into right and left portions.

SAGITTAL SECTION (SAJ-ih-tal SEK-shun): a cut (section) through the body dividing it into a right and left portion.

SALPINGECTOMY (sal-pin-JEK-to-me): removal of a fallopian (uterine) tube.

SALPINGITIS (al-pin-JI-tis): inflammation of a fallopian (uterine) tube.

SARCOIDOSIS (sahr-koi-DO-sis): chronic, progresssive, disorder of cells in connective tissue, spleen, liver, bone marrow, lungs, and lymph nodes. Small collections of cells (granulomas) form in affected organs and tissues.

SARCOMA (sar-KO-mah): cancerous (malignant) tumor of connective tissue, such as bone, muscle, fat, or cartilage.

SCAPULA (SKAP-u-lah): shoulder bone.

SCLERA (SKLE-rah): white, outer coat of the eyeball.

SCROTAL (SKRO-tal): pertaining to the scrotum.

SCROTUM (SKRO-tum): sac on the outside of the body that contains the testes.

SEBACEOUS GLAND (seh-BA-shus gland): oil (sebum)-producing gland in the skin.

SECTION (SEK-shun): an act of cutting; segment or subdivision of an organ.

SEIZURE (SE-zhur): a convulsion (involuntary contraction of muscles) or attack of EPILEPSY. A seizure can also indicate sudden attack or recurrence of a disease.

SELLA TURCICA (SEL-ah TUR-sih-ka): cup-like depression at the base of the skull; holds the pituitary gland.

SEMEN (SE-men): fluid composed of sperm cells and secretions from the prostate gland and other male exocrine glands.

SEMINOMA (sem-ih-NO-mah): malignant tumor of the testis.

SENSE ORGANS (sens OR-ganz): parts of the body that receive messages from the environment and relay them to the brain so that we see, hear, and feel sensations. Examples of sense organs are the eye, ear, and skin.

SEPTIC (SEP-tik): pertaining to infection.

SEPTICEMIA (sep-tih-SE-me-ah): infection in the blood. Septicemia is commonly called blood poisoning and is associated with the presence of bacteria or their poisons in the blood.

SHOCK (shok): group of symptoms (pale skin, rapid pulse, shallow breathing) that indicate poor oxygen supply to tissue and insufficient return of blood to the heart.

SIGMOID COLON (SIG-moyd KO-len): S-shaped lower portion of the colon.

SKIN (skin): outer covering that protects the body.

SKULL (skul): bone that surrounds the brain and other organs in the head.

SMALL INTESTINE (smal in-TES-tin): organ that receives food from the stomach; it is divided into three sections—duodenum, jejunum, and ileum.

SONOGRAM (SON-o-gram): record of sound waves after they bounce off organs in the body; an ULTRASOUND or echogram.

SPERMATOZOON (sper-mah-to-ZO-on): a sperm cell; pl. spermatozoa (sper-mah-to-ZO-ah).

SPINAL CAVITY (SPI-nal KAV-ih-te): space in the back that contains the spinal cord and is surrounded by the backbones.

SPINAL COLUMN (SPI-nal KOL-um): backbones; vertebrae.

SPINAL CORD (SPI-nal kord): bundle of nerves that extends from the brain down the back; carries electrical messages to and from the spinal cord.

SPINAL NERVES (SPI-nal nervz): nerves that transmit messages to and from the spinal cord.

SPLEEN (splen): organ in the left upper quadrant of the abdomen; stores blood cells and destroys red blood cells while producing white blood cells called LYMPHOCYTES.

SPLENOMEGALY (splehn-o-MEG-ah-le): enlargement of the spleen.

SPONDYLITIS (spon-dih-LI-tis): a chronic, serious inflammatory disorder of backbones involving erosion and collapse of vertebrae. See ANKYLOSING SPONDYLITIS.

SPONDYLOSIS (spon-dih-LO-sis): abnormal condition of a vertebra or vertebrae.

STERNUM (STER-num): breast bone.

STOMACH (STUM-ak): organ that receives food from the esophagus and sends it to the small intestine. Enzymes in the stomach breakdown food particles during digestion.

STOMATITIS (sto-mah-TI-tis): inflammation of the mouth.

STROKE (strok): Trauma to or blockage of blood vessels within the brain leading to less blood supply to brain tissue. This causes nerve cells in the brain to die and results in loss of function to the part of the body controlled by those nerve cells.

SUBCOSTAL (sub-KOS-tal): pertaining to below the ribs.

SUBCUTANEOUS TISSUE (sub-ku-TA-ne-us TIS-u): lower layer of the skin composed of fatty tissue.

SUBDURAL HEMATOMA (sub-DUR-al he-mah-TO-mah): collection of blood under the dura mater (outermost layer of the membranes surrounding the brain).

SUBGASTRIC (sub-GAS-trik): pertaining to below the stomach.

SUBHEPATIC (sub-heh-PAT-ik): pertaining to under the liver.

SUBSCAPULAR (sub-SKAP-u-lar): pertaining to under the shoulder bone.

SUBTOTAL (sub-TO-tal): less than total; just under the total amount.

SURGERY (SUR-jer-e): branch of medicine that treats disease by manual (hand) or operative methods.

SWEAT GLAND (sweht gland): organ in the skin that produces a watery substance containing salts.

SYNCOPE (SING-kah-pe): fainting; sudden loss of consciousness.

SYNDROME (SIN-drom): set of symptoms and signs of disease that occur together to indicate a disease condition.

SYSTEM (SIS-tem): group of organs working together to do a job in the body. For example, the digestive system includes the mouth, throat, stomach, and intestines, all of which help to bring food into the body, break it down, and deliver it to the bloodstream.

SYSTEMIC CIRCULATION (sis-TEM-ik ser-ku-LA-shun): the passage of blood from the heart to the tissues of the body and back to the heart.

TACHYCARDIA (tak-eh-KAR-de-ah): condition of fast, rapid heartbeat.

TACHYPNEA (tak-ip-NE-ah): condition of rapid breathing.

TENDON (TEN-don): connective tissue that joins muscles to bones.

TENDINITIS (ten-dih-NI-tis): inflammation of a tendon.

TENORRHAPHY (ten-OR-ah-fe): suture of a tendon.

TESTICLE (TES-tih-kl): see TESTIS.

TESTICULAR CARCINOMA (tes-TIK-u-lar kar-sih-NO-mah): malignant tumor orginating in a testis. An example of a testicular carcinoma is a seminoma.

TESTIS (TES-tis): one of two paired male organs in the scrotal sac. The testes (pl.) produce sperm cells and male hormone (testosterone); also called a testicle.

THORACENTESIS (tho-rah-sen-TE-sis): surgical puncture of the chest to remove fluid; thoracocentesis.

THORACIC (tho-RA-ik): pertaining to the chest.

THORACIC CAVITY (tho-RAS-ik KAV-ih-te): space above the abdomen, containing the heart, lungs, and other organs; the chest cavity.

THORACIC REGION (tho-RAS-ik RE-jin): backbones attached to the ribs and located in the region of the chest, between the neck and the waist.

THORACIC SURGEON (tho-RAS-ik SUR-jin): physician who operates on organs in the chest.

THORACIC VERTEBRA (tho-RAS-ik VER-teh-bra): a backbone in the region of the chest.

THORACOTOMY (tho-rah-KOT-o-me): incision of the chest.

THROAT (throt): see PHARYNX.

THROMBOCYTE (THROM-bo-sīt): clotting cell; a platelet.

THROMBOSIS (throm-BO-sis): abnormal condition of clot formation.

THROMBUS (THROM-bus): blood clot.

THYMOMA (thi-MO-mah): tumor (malignant) of the thymus gland.

THYMUS GLAND (THI-mus gland): endocrine gland in the middle of the chest that produces a hormone, *thymosin*. A much larger gland in children, the thymus aids the immune system by stimulating the production of white blood cells (lymphocytes).

THYROADENITIS (thi-ro-ah-de-NI-tis): inflammation of the thyroid gland.

THYROIDECTOMY (thi-roy-DEK-to-me): removal of the thyroid gland.

THYROID GLAND (THI-royd gland): endocrine gland in the neck that produces hormones, acting on cells all over the body. The hormones increase the activity of cells by stimulating metabolism and release of energy.

THYROXINE (thi-ROK-sin): hormone secreted by the thyroid gland; also known as T_4.

TIBIA (TIB-e-ah): larger of the two lower leg bones; shin bone.

TINNITUS (TIN-ih-tus): a noise in the ears, such as ringing, roaring, or buzzing.

TISSUE (TISH-u): groups of similar cells that work together to do a job in the body; muscle tissue, nerve tissue, and epithelial (skin) tissue.

TISSUE CAPILLARIES (TISH-u KAP-ih-lar-ez): tiny blood vessels that lie near cells and through whose walls gases, food, and waste materials pass.

TOMOGRAPHY (to-MOG-rah-fe): series of x-ray pictures that show an organ in depth by producing images of single tissue planes.

TONSILLECTOMY (ton-sih-LEK-to-me): removal (excision) of a tonsil or TONSILS.

TONSILS (TON-silz): lymphatic tissue in the back of the mouth near the throat.

TRACHEA (TRAY-ke-ah): tube that carries air from the throat to the BRONCHIAL TUBES; windpipe.

TRACHEOSTOMY (tray-ke-OS-to-me): opening of the trachea to the outside of the body.

TRACHEOTOMY (tray-ke-OT-o-me): incision of the trachea.

TRANSABDOMINAL (trans-ab-DOM-ih-nal): pertaining to across the abdomen.

TRANSGASTRIC (trans-GAS-trik): pertaining to across the stomach.

TRANSURETHRAL (tran-u-RE-thral): pertaining to across (through) the urethra. A *TURP* is a transurethral resection of the prostate by surgery through the urethra.

TRANSVERSE PLANE (trans-VERS plan): imaginary line that divides an organ or the body into an upper and lower portion; a cross-sectional view.

TRICUSPID VALVE (tri-KUS-pid valv): a fold of tissue between the upper and lower chambers on the right side of the heart. It has three cusps or points and prevents backflow of blood into the right ATRIUM when the heart is pumping blood.

TUBERCULOSIS (too-ber-ku-LO-sis): an infectious, inflammatory disease that commonly affects the lungs, although it can occur in any part of the body. It is caused by the tubercle bacillus (type of bacteria).

TYMPANIC MEMBRANE (tim-PAN-ik MEM-bran): see EARDRUM.

TYMPANOPLASTY (tim-pan-o-PLAS-te): surgical repair of the eardrum.

ULCER (UL-ser): sore or defect in the surface of an organ. Ulcers are produced by destruction of tissue.

ULCERATIVE COLITIS (ul-seh-RA-TIV ko-LI-tis): a recurrent disorder marked by ULCERS in the large bowel. Along with Crohn disease, this is an INFLAMMATORY BOWEL DISEASE with no known etiology (cause).

ULNA (UL-nah): one of two lower arm bones; on the little finger side of the hand.

ULTRASONOGRAPHY (ul-tra-son-OG-rah-fe): recording internal body structure using sound waves.

ULTRASOUND (UL-tra-sownd): sound waves with greater frequency than can be heard by the human ear. This energy is used to detect abnormalities by beaming the waves into the body and recording echoes that reflect off tissues.

UNILATERAL (u-nih-LAT-er-al): pertaining to one side.

UREA (u-RE-ah): chief nitrogen-containing waste that the kidney removes from the blood and elminates from the body in urine.

UREMIA (u-RE-me-ah): abnormal condition of excessive amounts of UREA in the bloodstream.

URETER (u-RE-ter or U-re-ter): one of two tubes that lead from the kidney to the urinary bladder.

URETERECTOMY (r-re-ter-EK-to-me): removal (excision) of a ureter.

URETHRA (u-RE-thrah): tube that carries urine from the urinary bladder to the outside of the body. In males, the urethra, which is within the penis, also carries sperm from the VAS DEFERENS to the outside of the body when sperm is discharged (ejaculation).

URETHRAL STRICTURE (u-RE-thral STRIK-shur): narrowing of the urethra.

URETHRITIS (u-re-THRI-tis): inflammation of the urethra.

URINALYSIS (u-rih-NAL-ih-sis): examination of urine to determine its contents.

URINARY BLADDER (UR-in-er-e BLA-der): muscular sac that holds urine and then releases it to leave the body through the urethra.

URINARY SYSTEM (UR-in-er-e SIS-tem): organs that produce and send urine out of the body. These organs are the kidneys, ureters, bladder, and urethra.

URINARY TRACT (UR-in-er-e trakt): tubes and organs that carry urine from the kidney to the outside of the body.

URINE (UR-in): fluid that is produced by the kidneys, passed through the ureters, stored in the bladder, and released from the body through the urethra.

UROLOGIST (u-ROL-o-jist): specialist in operating on the urinary tract in males and females and on the reproductive tract in males.

UROLOGY (u-ROL-o-je): study of the urinary system in males and females and the reproductive tract in males.

UTERINE (U-ter-in): pertaining to the uterus.

UTERINE TUBES (U-ter-in tubz): see FALLOPIAN TUBES.

UTERUS (U-ter-us): muscular organ in a female that holds and provides nourishment for the developing fetus; womb.

VAGINA (vah-JI-nah): muscular passageway from the uterus to the outside of the body.

VAGINITIS (vah-jih-NI-tis): inflammation of the vagina.

VARICOCELE (VAR-ih-ko-sel): swollen, twisted veins within the spermatic cord, above the testes. It produces a swelling in the scrotum that feels like a "bag of worms."

VARIX (VAH-riks): enlarged, swollen, tortuous veins; pl. varices (VAH-ri-sez).

VAS DEFERENS (vas DEHF-or-enz): one of two tubes that carry sperm from the testes to the urethra for ejaculation.

VASCULAR (VAS-ku-lar): pertaining to blood vessels.

VASCULITIS (vas-ku-LI-tis): inflammation of blood vessels.

VASECTOMY (vas-EK-to-me): removal of the vas deferens or a portion of it so that sperm cells are prevented from becoming part of SEMEN.

VASOCONSTRICTOR (vas-o-kon-STRIK-tor): drug that narrows blood vessels, especially small arteries.

VEIN (van): blood vessel that carries blood back to the heart from tissues of the body.

VENTRICLE (VEN-tri-kl): one of the two lower chambers of the heart. The right ventricle receives blood from the right atrium (upper chamber) and sends it to the lungs. The left ventricle receives blood from the left atrium and sends it to the body through the aorta.

VENULE (VEN-ul): small vein.

VENULITIS (ven-u-LI-tis): inflammation of a small vein.

VERTEBRA (VER-teh-brah): a backbone.

VERTEBRAE (VER-teh-bray): backbones.

VERTEBRAL (VER-teh-bral): pertaining to a backbone.

VESICAL (VES-ih-kal): pertaining to the urinary bladder (VESIC/O).

VIRUS (VI-rus): small infectious agent that can reproduce itself only when it is inside another living cell (host).

WOMB (woom): see UTERUS.

Glossary of Word Parts

Section I of this glossary is a list of **medical terminology** word parts and their **English** meanings. Section II is the reverse of that list, giving **English** meanings and their corresponding **medical terminology** word parts.

SECTION I: MEDICAL TERMINOLOGY → ENGLISH

Word Part	Meaning
a-, an-	no, not
ab-	away from
abdomin/o	abdomen
-ac	pertaining to
ad-	toward
aden/o	gland
adren/o	adrenal gland
-al	pertaining to
-algia	pain
alveol/o	alveolus (air sac within the lung)
amni/o	amnion (sac that surrounds the embryo)
-an	pertaining to
ana-	up, apart
an/o	anus
angi/o	vessel (blood)
ante-	before, forward
anti-	against
append/o, appendic/o	appendix
-ar	pertaining to
arteri/o	artery
arteriol/o	small artery
arthr/o	joint
-ary	pertaining to
-ation	process, condition
axill/o	armpit
balan/o	penis
bi-	two
bi/o	life
brady-	slow
bronch/o	bronchial tube
bronchiol/o	small bronchial tube

Word Part	Meaning
calcane/o	calcaneus (heel bone)
capillar/o	capillary
carcin/o	cancer, cancerous
cardi/o	heart
carp/o	wrist bones (carpals)
-cele	hernia
-centesis	surgical puncture to remove fluid
cephal/o	head
cerebell/o	cerebellum (posterior part of the brain)
cerebr/o	cerebrum (largest part of the brain)
cervic/o	neck
chem/o	drug, chemical
cholecyst/o	gallbladder
choledoch/o	common bile duct
chondr/o	cartilage
chron/o	time
-cision	process of cutting
cis/o	to cut
clavicul/o	clavicle (collar bone)
-coccus	berry-shaped bacteria (pl. cocci)
coccyg/o	tailbone
col/o	colon (large intestine)
colon/o	colon
colp/o	vagina
comi/o	to care for
con-	with, together
coni/o	dust
-coniosis	abnormal condition of dust
coron/o	heart
cost/o	rib
crani/o	skull
crin/o	secrete
-crine	secretion
-crit	separate
cry/o	cold
cutane/o	skin
cyst/o	urinary bladder
cyt/o	cell
-cyte	cell
dermat/o, derm/o	skin
dia-	through, complete

Word Part	Meaning
dur/o	dura mater (outermost meningeal layer)
dys-	painful, abnormal, bad, difficult
-eal	pertaining to
ec-	out, outside
ecto-	out, outside
-ectomy	excision (resection, removal)
-emesis	vomiting
-emia	blood condition
en-	within, in, inner
encephal/o	brain
endo-	within, in, inner
endocrin/o	endocrine glands
endometri/o	endometrium (inner lining of the uterus)
enter/o	intestines (usually small intestine)
epi-	above, upon
epiglott/o	epiglottis
epitheli/o	skin (surface tissue)
erythr/o	red
esophag/o	esophagus
esthesi/o	sensation
ex-, extra-	out, outside
femor/o	femur, thigh bone
fibul/o	fibula (smaller lower leg bone)
gastr/o	stomach
gen/o	to produce
-gen	to produce
-genesis	producing, forming
-genic	pertaining to producing, produced by
ger/o	old age
glyc/o	sugar
gnos/o	knowledge
-gram	record
-graphy	process of recording, to record
gynec/o	woman, female
hemat/o, hem/o	blood
hepat/o	liver
humer/o	humerus (upper arm bone)

Word Part	Meaning
hyper-	excessive, above
hypo-	below, deficient
hypophys/o	pituitary gland
hyster/o	uterus
-ia	condition
iatr/o	treatment
-ic	pertaining to
ile/o	ileum (third part of small intestine)
ili/o	ilium (upper part of hip bone)
in-	in, into
-ine	pertaining to
inguin/o	groin
inter-	between
intra-	within
-ior	pertaining to
isch/o	to hold back
-ism	condition, process
-ist	specialist
-itis	inflammation
lapar/o	abdomen
laryng/o	larynx (voice box)
later/o	side
leuk/o	white
-listhesis	to slip, slide
lith/o	stone
-lith	stone
-logy	study of
lumb/o	loin, waist region
lymph/o	lymph
lymphaden/o	lymph nodes
lymphangi/o	lymph vessel
lys/o	separation, breakdown, destruction
-lysis	separation, breakdown, destruction
mal-	bad
mamm/o	breast
mast/o	breast
mediastin/o	mediastinum
medull/o	medulla oblongata (lower part of the brain)

Word Part	Meaning
-megaly	enlargement
men/o	menstruation
mening/o	meninges (membranes covering brain and spinal cord)
meta-	beyond, change
metacarp/o	metacarpals (hand bones)
metatars/o	metatarsals (foot bones)
metr/o	uterus; to measure
-metry	measurement
-mortem	death
-motor	movement
muscul/o	muscle
my/o	muscle
myel/o	bone marrow (with -blast, -oma, -cyte, -genic)
myel/o	spinal cord (with -gram, -itis, -cele)
myos/o	muscle
myring/o	eardrum
nas/o	nose
nat/i	birth
neo-	new
nephr/o	kidney
neur/o	nerve
nos/o	disease
obstetr/o	midwife
ocul/o	eye
-oma	tumor, mass, swelling
onc/o	tumor
oophor/o	ovary
ophthalm/o	eye
-opsy	process of viewing
opt/o	eye
or/o	mouth
orch/o	testicle, testis
orchi/o	testicle, testis
orchid/o	testicle, testis
orth/o	straight
-osis	abnormal condition
oste/o	bone
ot/o	ear
-ous	pertaining to
ovari/o	ovary

Word Part	Meaning
pancreat/o	pancreas
para-	beside, near, along the side of
-partum	birth
path/o	disease
-pathy	disease condition
ped/o	child
pelv/o	hip bone
per-	through
peri-	surrounding
peritone/o	peritoneum (membrane around abdominal organs)
perone/o	fibula
-pexy	fixation (surgical)
phalang/o	phalanges (finger and toe bones)
pharyng/o	pharynx, throat
-philia	attraction to
phleb/o	vein
phren/o	diaphragm
phren/o	mind
plas/o	formation, growth, development
-plasm	formation, growth, development
-plasty	surgical repair
-plegia	paralysis
pleur/o	pleura (membranes surrounding the lungs)
-pnea	breathing
pneum/o	air, lung
pneumon/o	lung
-poiesis	formation
post-	after, behind
pre-	before
pro-, pros-	before, forward
proct/o	anus and rectum
prostat/o	prostate gland
psych/o	mind
-ptosis	prolapse, sagging
-ptysis	spitting
pulmon/o	lung
pyel/o	renal pelvis (central section of the kidney)
radi/o	x-ray; radius (lateral lower arm bone)
re-, retro-	behind, back
rect/o	rectum
ren/o	kidney
retin/o	retina of the eye

Word Part	Meaning
rheumat/o	flow, fluid
rhin/o	nose
-rrhage	bursting forth of blood
-rrhagia	bursting forth of blood
-rrhea	flow, discharge
sacr/o	sacrum
salping/o	fallopian (uterine) tube; eustachian tube
-salpinx	fallopian (uterine) tube; eustachian tube
sarc/o	flesh
scapul/o	shoulder blade (bone)
-sclerosis	condition of hardening
-scope	instrument to view or visually examine
-scopy	process of viewing or visual examination
scrot/o	scrotal sac, scrotum
-section	to cut
-sept/o	infection
septic/o	infection
-sis	condition
-somatic	pertaining to the body
son/o	sound
-spasm	constriction
spin/o	backbone
splen/o	spleen
spondyl/o	vertebra, backbone
-stasis	stop, control; place, to stand
-stat	stop, control
stern/o	sternum (breast bone)
-stomy	opening
sub-	under, below
sym-	with, together (use before b, p, and m)
syn-	with, together
tachy-	fast
-tension	pressure
theli/o	nipple
-therapy	treatment
-thesis	to put or place
thorac/o	chest
thromb/o	clot
thym/o	thymus gland
thyr/o, thyroid/o	thyroid gland

Word Part	Meaning
tib/o	tibia or shin bone (larger lower leg bone)
-tic	pertaining to
-tomy	incision, process of cutting
tonsill/o	tonsils
top/o	to put, place
trache/o	trachea (windpipe)
trans-	across, through
tri-	three
troph/o	development, nourishment
-trophy	development, nourishment
tympan/o	eardrum
uln/o	ulna (medial lower arm bone)
ultra-	beyond
-um	structure
uni-	one
ureter/o	ureter
urethr/o	urethra
ur/o	urine, urinary tract
-uria	urine condition
uter/o	uterus
vagin/o	vagina
vas/o	vessel, vas deferens
vascul/o	blood vessel
ven/o	vein
vertebr/o	vertebra (backbone)
vesic/o	urinary bladder
-y	condition; process

SECTION II: ENGLISH → MEDICAL TERMINOLOGY

Meaning	Word Part
abdomen	abdomin/o (use with -al, -centesis)
	lapar/o (use with -scope, -scopy, -tomy)
abnormal	dys-
abnormal condition	-osis
above	epi-, hyper-
across	trans-
adrenal gland	adren/o
after	post-
against	anti-
air	pneum/o
air sac	alveol/o
along the side of	para-
alveolus	alveol/o
amnion	amni/o
anus	an/o
anus and rectum	proct/o
apart	ana-
appendix	append/o (use with -ectomy)
	appendic/o (use with -itis)
armpit	axill/o
artery	arteri/o
attraction to	-philia
away from	ab-
backbone	spin/o (use with -al)
	spondyl/o (use with -itis, -listhesis, -osis, -pathy)
	vertebr/o (use with -al)
bacteria (berry-shaped)	-coccus (pl. -cocci)
bad	dys-, mal-
before	ante-, pre-, pro-, pros-
behind	post-, re-, retro-
below	hypo-, sub-
beside	para-
between	inter-
beyond	meta-, ultra-
birth	nat/i, -partum
bladder (urinary)	cyst/o (use with -ic, -itis, -cele, -gram, -scopy)
	vesic/o (use with -al, -stomy, -tomy)

Meaning	Word Part
blood	hem/o (use with -cyte, -dialysis, -globin, -lysis, -philia, -ptysis, -rrhage, -stasis, -stat)
	hemat/o (use with -crit, -emesis, -logist, -logy, -oma, -poiesis, -salpinx, -uria)
blood condition	-emia
blood vessel	angi/o (use with -ectomy, -dysplasia, -genesis, -gram, -graphy, -oma, -plasty, -spasm)
	vas/o (use with -constriction, -dilatation, -motor)
	vascul/o (use with -ar, -itis)
body	-somatic
bone	oste/o
bone marrow	myel/o
brain	encephal/o
breakdown	-lysis, lys/o
breast	mamm/o (use with -ary, -gram, -graphy, -plasty)
	mast/o (use with -algia, -ectomy, -itis)
breast bone	stern/o
breathing	-pnea
bronchial tube	bronch/o
bronchiole	bronchiol/o
bursting forth of blood	-rrhage, -rrhagia
calcaneus	calcane/o
cancer	carcin/o
cancerous	carcin/o
capillary	capillar/o
care for (to)	comi/o
carpals	carp/o
cartilage	chondr/o
cell	-cyte, cyt/o
cerebellum	cerebell/o
cerebrum	cerebr/o
change	meta-
chemical	chem/o
chest	thorac/o
child	ped/o
clavicle	clavicul/o
clot	thromb/o
cold	cry/o
collarbone	clavicul/o
colon	col/o (use with -ectomy, -itis, -stomy)
	colon/o (use with -pathy, -scope, -scopy)

Meaning	Word Part
common bile duct	choledoch/o
complete	dia-
condition	-ation, -ia, -ism, -osis, -sis, -y
constriction	-spasm
control	-stasis, -stat
cut	-cision, cis/o, -section, -tomy
death	-mortem, necr/o
deficient	hypo-
destroy	lys/o, -lysis
development	troph/o, -trophy
diaphragm	phren/o
difficult	dys-
discharge	-rrhea
disease	path/o, -pathy; nos/o
drug	chem/o
dura mater	dur/o
dust	coni/o
dust condition	-coniosis
ear	ot/o
eardrum	myring/o (use with -ectomy, -itis, -tomy)
	tympan/o (use with -ic, -metry, -plasty)
electricity	electr/o
endocrine gland	endocrin/o
endometrium	endometr/o
enlargement	-megaly
epiglottis	epiglott/o
esophagus	esophag/o
eustachian tube	salping/o
excessive	hyper-
eye	ocul/o (use with -ar, -facial, -motor)
	ophthalm/o (use with -ia, -ic, -logist, -logy, -pathy, -plasty, -plegia, -scope, -scopy)
	opt/o (use with -ic, -metrist)
fallopian tube	salping/o, -salpinx
fast	tachy-
female	gynec/o
femur	femor/o

Meaning	Word Part
fibula	fibul/o, perone/o
fixation (surgical)	-pexy
flesh	sarc/o
flow	-rrhea
fluid	rheumat/o
foot bones	metatars/o
formation	plas/o, -plasm, -poiesis, -genesis
forward	ante-, pro-, pros-
gallbladder	cholecyst/o
gland	aden/o
groin	inguin/o
growth	plas/o, -plasm
hand bones	metacarp/o
hardening	-sclerosis
head	cephal/o
heart	cardi/o (use with -ac, -graphy, -logy, -logist, -megaly, -pathy, -vascular)
	coron/o (use with -ary)
heel bone	calcane/o
hernia	-cele
hip bone	pelv/o
hold back	isch/o
humerus	humer/o
ileum	ile/o
ilium	ili/o
in, into	in-, en-
incision	-tomy, -section
infection	sept/o, septic/o
inflammation	-itis
inner	endo-
instrument to record	-graph
instrument to view	-scope
intestines (small)	enter/o
joint	arthr/o

Meaning	Word Part
kidney	nephr/o (use with -algia, -ectomy, -ic, -itis, -lith, -megaly, -oma, -osis, -pathy, -ptosis, -sclerosis, -stomy, -tomy)
	ren/o (use with -al, -gram)
kidney (central section)	pyel/o
knowledge	gnos/o
larynx	laryng/o
life	bi/o
liver	hepat/o
loin	lumb/o
lung	pneum/o (use with -coccus, -coniosis)
	pneumon/o (use with -ectomy, -ia, -ic, -itis, -pathy, -therapy, -thorax)
	pulmon/o (use with -ary)
lymph	lymph/o
lymph node	lymphaden/o
lymph vessel	lymphangi/o
mass	-oma
measure	metr/o, -meter, -metry
mediastinum	mediastin/o
medulla oblongata	medull/o
meninges	mening/o
menstruation	men/o
metacarpals	metacarp/o
metatarsals	metatars/o
midwife	obstetr/o
mind	psych/o
mouth	or/o (use with -al)
	stomat/o (use with -itis)
movement	-motor
muscle	muscul/o (use with -ar, -skeletal)
	myos/o (use with -itis)
	my/o (use with -algia, -ectomy, -oma, -gram, -neural)
near	para-
neck	cervic/o
nerve	neur/o
new	neo-

Meaning	Word Part
nipple	theli/o
no, not	a-, an-
nose	nas/o (use with -al)
	rhin/o (use with -itis, -rrhea, -plasty)
nourishment	troph/o, -trophy
old age	ger/o
one	uni-
opening	-stomy
out, outside	ec-, ecto-, ex-, extra-
ovary	oophor/o (use with -itis, -ectomy, -pexy, -plasty, -tomy)
	ovari/o (use with -an)
pain	-algia
painful	dys-
pancreas	pancreat/o
paralysis	-plegia
pelvis	pelv/o
pelvis (renal)	pyel/o
penis	balan/o
peritoneum	peritone/o
pertaining to	-ac, -al, -an, -ar, -ary, -eal, -ic, -ine, -ior, -ous, -tic
phalanges	phalang/o
pharynx	pharyng/o
pituitary gland	hypophys/o
place	top/o; -stasis
pleura	pleur/o
pressure	-tension
process	-ation, -ism, -y
process of cutting	-cision, -tomy, -section
process of recording	-graphy
process of viewing	-opsy, -scopy
produce (to)	-gen, gen/o
produced by	-genic
producing	-genic, -genesis
prolapse	-ptosis
prostate gland	prostat/o
puncture to remove fluid	-centesis

Meaning	Word Part
put, place	top/o, -thesis
radius (lower arm bone)	radi/o
record	-gram
recording (process)	-graphy
rectum	rect/o
red	erythr/o
repair	-plasty
retina	retin/o
rib	cost/o
sacrum	sacr/o
sagging	-ptosis
scapula	scapul/o
scrotum	scrot/o
secrete, secretion	-crine, crin/o
sensation	esthesi/o
separation	-crit, -lysis
shin bone	tibi/o
shoulder blade	scapul/o
side	later/o
skin	cutane/o (use with -ous)
	derm/o, (use with -al) dermat/o (use with -itis, -logy, -osis)
	epitheli/o (use with -al)
skull	crani/o
slip (to)	-listhesis
slow	brady-
small artery	arteri/o
small intestine	enter/o
sound	son/o
specialist	-ist
spinal cord	myel/o
spine	spin/o
spitting	-ptysis
spleen	splen/o
stand (to)	-stasis
sternum	stern/o
stomach	gastr/o
stone	lith/o, -lith
stop	-stasis, -stat

Meaning	Word Part
straight	orth/o
structure	-um
study of	-logy
sugar	glyc/o
surgical puncture to remove fluid	-centesis
surgical repair	-plasty
surrounding	peri-
swelling	-oma
tailbone	coccyg/o
testicle, testis	orch/o, orchi/o, orchid/o
thigh bone	femor/o
throat	pharyng/o
three	tri-
through	dia-, per-, trans-
thymus gland	thym/o
thyroid gland	thyr/o, thyroid/o
tibia	tibi/o
time	chron/o
together	con-, syn-
tonsil	tonsill/o
trachea	trache/o
treatment	iatr/o, -therapy
tumor	onc/o, -oma
two	bi-
under	hypo-, sub-
up	ana-
upon	epi-
ureter	ureter/o
urethra	urethr/o
urinary bladder	cyst/o, vesic/o
urinary tract	ur/o
urine	ur/o
urine condition	-uria
uterine tube	salping/o
uterus	hyster/o (use with -ectomy, -graphy, -gram)
	metr/o (use with -itis, -rrhagia)
	uter/o (use with -ine)
uterus (inner lining)	endometr/o, endometri/o

Meaning	Word Part
vagina	colp/o (use with -pexy, -plasty, -scope, -scopy, -tomy)
	vagin/o (use with -al, -itis)
vas deferens	vas/o
vein	phleb/o (use with -ectomy, -itis, -lith, -thrombosis, -tomy)
	ven/o (use with -ous, -gram)
vertebra	spin/o (use with -al)
	spondyl/o (use with -itis, -listhesis, -osis, -pathy)
	vertebr/o (use with -al)
vessel	angi/o (use with -ectomy, -dysplasia, -genesis, -gram, -graphy, -oma, -plasty, -spasm)
	vas/o (use with -constriction, -dilatation, -motor)
	vascul/o (use with -ar, -itis)
view (to)	-opsy
visual examination	-scopy
voice box	laryng/o
waist region	lumb/o
white	leuk/o
windpipe	trache/o
with	con-, syn-
within	en-, endo-, intra-
woman	gynec/o
wrist bones	carp/o
x-ray	radi/o

Glossary of English → Spanish Terms

GLOSSARY OF ENGLISH → SPANISH TERMS

Here is a list of English → Spanish terms that will help you communicate with Spanish-speaking patients in offices, hospitals, and other medical settings. It includes parts of the body and other medical terms as well.

abdomen	abdomen (**AHB**-doh-mehn)
acne	acné (ahk-**NEH**)
acoustic	acustico (ah-**KOOS**-tee-ko)
adenoid	adenoide (ah-deh-**NOH**-ee-deh)
amebic	amébico (ah-**MEH**-bee-ko)
analgesic	analgesicos (ah-nahl-**HEH**-see-kohs)
anemia	anemia (ah-**NEH**-mee-ah)
anesthesia	anestesia (ah-nehs-**TEH**-see-ah)
angina	angina (ahn-**HEE**-na)
angioma	angioma (ahn-hee-**OH**-ma)
ankle	tobillo (toh-**BEE**-yo)
antacid	antiácidos (ahn-tee-**AH**-see-dohs)
antiarrhythmic	antiarritmias (ahn-tee-ah-**REEHT**-mee-ahs)
antibiotic	antibiótico (ahn-tee-bee-**OH**-tee-ko)
anticonvulsant	anticonvulsivo (ahn-tee-kohn-**BOOL**-see-bo)
antidiarrheal	antidiarrea (ahn-tee-dee-ah-**RREH**-ah)
antiemetic	antiemético (ahn-tee-eh-**MEH**-tee-ko)
antiepileptic	antiepileptico (ahn-tee-eh-pee-**LEHP**-tee-ko)
antihistamine	antihistamínico (ahn-tee-ees-tah-**MEE**-nee-ko)
antiviral	antivirus (ahn-tee-**BEE**-roos)
anus	ano (**AH**-no)
appendix	apéndice (ah-**PEHN**-dees)
armpit	axila (ahx-**EE**-la)
arteriogram	arteriograma (ahr-teh-ree-oh-**GRAH**-ma)
arthritis	artritis (ahr-**TREE**-tees)
asthma	asma (**AHS**-mah)
bacteria	bacteria (bahk-**TEH**-ree-ah)
barbiturates	barbitúricos (bahr-bee-**TOO**-ree-kohs)
birthmark	lunares (loo-**NAH**-rehs)
bleeding	sangrado (sahn-**GRAH**-do)
blood	sangre (**SAHN**-greh)
blood count	biometría hemática (bee-oh-meh-**TREE**-ah eh-**MAH**-tee-kah)
bradycardia	bradicardia (brah-dee-**KAHR**-dee-ah)
brain	cerebro (se-**RE**-bro)
breast/chest	seno (**SEH**-noh), pecho (**PEH**-choh)
bronchial tube	bronquio (**BROHN**-kjo)
bronchitis	bronquitis (brohn-**KEE**-tees)

bruises	moretones (moh-reh-**TOH**-nehs)
burn	quemadura (ke-mah-**DU**-ra)
calf	pantorrilla (pan-to-**REE**-ya)
callus	callo (**KAH**-yo)
calm	calma (**KAHL**-mah)
cardiac	cardiaco (kahr-dee-**AH**-ko)
cataract	catarata (kah-tah-**RAH**-ta)
cervix	cuello uterino (**KWE**-yo oo-teh-**REE**-noh), cerviz (**SER**-vees)
chancre	chancro (**CHAHN**-kroh)
cheek	mejilla (meh-**HI**-ya)
chemotherapy	quimioterapia (kee-mee-oh-teh-**RAH**-pee-ah)
chin	barbilla (bar-**BEE**-ya), menton (**MEN**-ton)
cholesterol	colesterol (koh-**LEHS**-teh-rohl)
cirrhosis	cirrosis (see-**RROH**-sees)
claustrophobia	claustrofobia (klah-oos-troh-**FOH**-bee-ah)
coagulation	coagulacion (koh-ah-goo-**LAH**-see-ohn)
collar bone	clavícula (klah-**VEE**-kuh-la)
colon	colon (**KOH**-lohn)
constipation	estrñimiento (ehs-treh-nyee-mee-**EHN**-to)
cortisone	cortisona (kohr-tee-**SOHN**-ah)
cough	tos (tohs)
cyanotic	cianótico (see-ah-**NOH**-tee-ko)
decongestants	decongestionantes (dehs-kohn-hehs-tee-oh-**MAHN**-tehs)
dehydrated	deshidratado (deh-see-drah-**TAH**-do)
delirious	delirio (deh-**LEE**-ree-oh)
depressed	deprimido (deh-pree-**MEE**-do)
diabetes	diabetes (dee-ah-**BEH**-tees)
diarrhea	diarrea (dee-ah-**RREH**-ah)
digitalis	digitales (dee-hee-**TAH**-lehs)
ear (inner)	oído (o-**EE**-do)
ear (outer)	oreja (or-**EH**-ha)
ecchymosis	equimosis (eh-kee-**MOH**-sees)
eczema	eccema (**EHK**-seh-ma)
elbow	codo (**KOH**-do)
embolism	embolismo (ehm-bohl-**EES**-mo)
emetic	emético (eh-**MEH**-tee-ko)
enteritis	enteritis (ehn-teh-**REE**-tees)
epilepsy	epilepsia (eh-pee-**LEHP**-see-ah)
euphoric	eufórico (eh-oo-**FOH**-ree-ko)
exudate	exudado (ehx-oo-**DAH**-do)
eye	ojo (**O**-ho)
eyebrow	ceja (**SEH**-ha)

eyelash	pestaña (pes-**TA**-nya)
eyelids	párpados (**PAR**-pa-dos)
fibroid	fibroide (fee-**BROH**-ee-deh)
finger	dedo (**DEH**-do)
fingernail	úna (**OO**-nya)
fist	púno (**POO**-nyoh)
fistula	fistula (**FEES**-too-la)
foot	pie (**PEE**-eh)
forearm	antebrazo (an-teh-**BRAH**-zo)
forehead	frente (**FREN**-teh)
fungus	hongos (**OHN**-gohs)
gallbladder	vesícula biliar (ves-**EE**-ku-lah bee-**LEE**-ahr)
gangrene	gangrena (gahn-**GREH**-na)
gastroenteritis	gastroenteritis (gahs-troh-ehn-teh-**REE**-tees)
gastroenterology	gastroenterología (gahs-troh-ehn-teh-roh-**LOH**-'gee-ah)
genital organs	organos genitales (orh-**GAH**-nos heh-nee-**TAH**-lehs)
glaucoma	glaucoma (glaw-**KO**-ma)
groin	ingle (**EEN**-gleh)
gums	encías (en-**SEE**-as)
gynecologist	ginecólogo (hee-neh-**KOH**-loh-go)
hair	cabello (kah-**BE**-yo), pelo (**PEH**-lo)
hand	mano (mah-no)
heart	corazón (ko-rah-**ZOHN**)
hematology	hematología (eh-mah-toh-loh-**HEE**-ah)
hematoma	hematoma (eh-mah-**TOH**-ma)
hemolysis	hemólisis (eh-**MOH**-lee-sees)
hemorrhage	hemorragia (eh-moh-**RAH**-hee-ah)
hepatitis	hepatitis (eh-pah-**TEE**-tees)
hernia	hernia (**EHR**-nee-ah)
hip	cadera (kah-**DEH**-ra)
hypertension	hipertensión (ee-pehr-tehn-see-**OHN**)
icteric	ictérico (eek-**TEH**-ree-ko)
infection	infección (een-fehk-see-**OHN**)
inflammation	inflamación (een-flah-mah-see-**OHN**)
insulin	insulina (een-soo-**LEE**-na)
intestine	intestino (een-**TES**-tee-no)
intramuscular	intramuscular (een-trah-**MOOS**-koo-lahr)
intravenous	intravenoso (een-trah-beh-**NOH**-so)
irradiate	irradiar (ee-**RAH**-dee-ahr)
jaw	quijada (koo-ee-**HA**-da), mandíbula (man-**DEE**-boo-la)

kidney	riñón (ree-**NOHN**)
knee	rodilla (ro-**DEE**-ya)
laparoscopy	laparoscopia (lah-pah-rahs-**KOH**-pee-ah)
laryngitis	laringitis (lah-reen-**HEE**-tee)
laxative	laxante (lahx-**AHN**-teh)
left	izquierdo(a) (ees-kee-**EHR**-doh [dah])
leg	pierna (pee-**EHR**-na)
ligament	ligamento (lee-gah-**MEHN**-to)
lingual	lingual (leen-**GOO**-ahl)
lip	labio (**LAH**-bee-o)
lithium	litio (**LEE**-tee-oh)
liver	hígado (**EEH**-gah-do)
low cholesterol	poco colesterol (**POH**-koh koh-**LEHS**-teh-rhol)
low fat	poco grasa (**POH**-koh **GRAH**-sa)
low sodium	poco sal (**POH**-koh sahl)
lung	pulmon (pool-**MOHN**)
meningitis	meningitis (meh-neen-**HEE**-tees)
morphine	morfina (mohr-**FEE**-na)
mouth	boca (**BOH**-ka)
muscle	músculo (**MOOS**-koo-lo)
narcotics	narcóticos (nahr-**KOH**-tee-kohs)
nasal	nasal (**NAH**-sahl)
nausea	náusea (**NAH**-oo-seh-ah)
navel	ombligo (om-**BLI**-go)
neck	cuello (koo-**EH**-yo)
neonatal	neonatal (neh-oh-**NAH**-tahl)
nephrology	especialista en los riñónes (ehs-peh-see-ah-**LEES**-tah en los ree-**NYO**-nes)
nervous	nervioso (ner-bee-**OH**-so)
neurotic	neurótico (new-**RO**-tee-ko)
nipple	pezón (peh-**ZON**)
nitroglycerin	nitroglicerina (nee-troh-glee-seh-**REE**-na)
nose	nariz (na-**RIZ**)
nostrils	fosas nasales (**FOH**-sas na-**SA**-les)
Novocain	novocaína (noh-boh-kah-**EE**-nah)
nuclear medicine	medicina nuclear (meh-dee-**SEE**-nah **NOO**-kleh-ahr)
obstetrics	obstetriz (ohb-**STEH**-'trees)
oncology	oncología (ohn-koh-loh-'hee-ah)
ophthalmic	oftálmico (ohf-**TAHL**-mee-ko)
ophthalmology	oftalmólogo (ohf-**TAHL**-'moh-loh-goh)

orthopedics	cirujano ortopédico (see-roo-'hah-noh ohr-toh-'peh-dee-koh)
otic	otico (**OH**-ti-co)
ovary	ovario (oh-**VAH**-ree-oh)
palate	paladar (pah-lah-**DAR**)
palpation	palpación (pahl-pah-see-**OHN**)
palpitation	palpitación (pahl-pee-tah-see-**OHN**)
pancreas	páncreas (**PAHN**-kre-as)
pancreatitis	pancreatitis (pahn-kreh-ah-**TEE**-tees)
paralytic	paralitico (pah-rah-**LEE**-tee-ko)
pathogen	patogénico (pah-toh-**HEH**-nee-ko)
pathological	patológico (pah-toh-**LOH**-hee-ko)
pathology	patológia (pah-toh-**LOH**-hee-ah)
pediatrics	pediatra (peh-dee-'**AH**-trah)
pelvis	pelvis (**PEL**-vees)
penis	pene (**PEH**-neh), miembro (mee-**EHM**-bro)
pneumonia	pulmonía/neumonía (pool-moh-**NEE**-ah/neh-oo-moh-**NEE**-ah)
pruritic	pruritico (proo-**REE**-tee-ko)
psychiatry	psiquiatra (see-kee-'**AH**-trah)
psychologist	psicólogo (see-'koh-loh-goh)
psoriasis	soriasis (soh-ree-**AH**-sees)
pubic	púbico (**POO**-bee-ko)
pyorrhea	piorrea (pee-**OH**-rreh-ah)
radiology	radiólogo (rah-dee-'oh-loh-goh)
rectum	recto (**REHK**-to)
rheumatic	reumático (reh-oo-**MAH**-tee-ko)
rib	costilla (kos-**TEE**-ya)
right	derecho(a) (deh-**REH**-choh [chah])
roseola	roseóla (roh-seh-**OH**-la)
rubella	rubeóla (roo-beh-**OH**-la)
scalp	cuero cabelludo (**KWE**-ro ka-beh-**YU**-do)
sebaceous	sebáceo (seh-**BAH**-seh-oh)
sedatives	sedativo/sedantes (seh-**DAH**-tee-boh/seh-**DAHN**-tehs)
shin	espinilla (ees-pih-**NEE**-ya)
shoulder	hombro (**OHM**-bro)
skin	piel (pee-**EL**)
skull	craneo (kra-**NEH**-oh)
spinal column	columna vertebral (koh-**LUHM**-nah ber-**TE**-brahl)
spleen	bazo (**BAH**-zoh), esplin (**EHS**-pleen)
stethoscope	estetoscópio (ehs-teh-tohs-**KOH**-pee-oh)
stomach	estómago (es-**TOH**-mah-go)
stool sample	muestra de excremento (moo-**EHS**-trah deh ehx-kreh-**MENH**-to)
subaxillary	subaxilar (soob-**AHX**-ee-lahr)

subcutaneous	subcutáneo (soob-koo-**TAH**-neh-oh)
sublingual	sublingual (soob-**LEEN**-goo-al)
substernal	subesternal (soob-ehs-**TEHR**-nal)
surgeon	cirujano (see-roo-**HA**-noh)
surgery	cirugía (see-roo-**HEE**-ah)
symptoms	síntomas (**SEEN**-toh-mas)
syncope	sincope (**SEEN**-koh-peh)
systole	sístole (**SEES**-toh-leh)
teeth	dientes (dee-**EN**-tes)
temple	sein (**SE**-en)
testicles	testículos (tes-**TEE**-ku-los)
tetanus	tétano (**TEH**-tah-noh)
therapy	terapia (teh-**RAH**-pee-ah)
thigh	muslo (**MOO**-sloh)
throat	garganta (gahr-**GAHN**-ta)
thyroid	tiroides/tiroidea (tee-**ROH**-ee-dehs/tee-roh-**EE**-deh-ah)
toes	dedos (**DEH**-dos)
tongue	lengua (**LEN**-goo-ah)
tonsillitis	tonsilitis/amigdalitis (tohn-see-**LEE**-tees/ah-meeg-dah-**LEE**-tees)
tonsils	amígdalas (ah-**MEEG**-da-las)
ulcer	úlcera (**OOL**-seh-ra)
ulnar	ulnar (**OOL**-nahr)
ultrasound	ultrasonido (ool-trah-soh-**NEE**-do)
uremia	uremia (oo-**REH**-mee-ah)
urinary bladder	vejiga (veh-**HEE**-ga)
urine	orina (oh-**REE**-na)
urticaria	uritcaria (oor-tee-**KAH**-ree-ah)
uterus	útero (**OO**-teh-roh), matriz (**MAHT**-reez)
uvula	úvula (**OO**-boo-lah)
vaginitis	vaginitis (bah-hee-**NEE**-tees)
vagus	vago (**BAH**-goh)
valve	válvula (**BAL**-bu-la)
varicocele	varicocéle (bah-ree-koh-**SEH**-leh)
vertigo	vértigo (**BER**-ti-go)
waist	cintura (sin-**TU**-ra)
womb	vientre (bjen-tre)
wrist	muñeca (mu-**NYE**-kah)
x-rays	rayos equis (**RAH**-yohs **EH**-kiss)
zygomatic	cigomático (see-go-**MAH**-tee-ko)

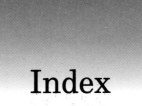

Index

Note: Page numbers in *italics* indicate figures; page numbers followed by t indicate tables.